Conquering Obesity, Conquering Mountains

6 Steps to Fail-Proof, Sustainable
Weight Loss and a Healthy Lifestyle
Through a Holistic System

Bruce Fam • Coach Aizat • Praveen Raj

Authors: Bruce Fam, Coach Aizat & Praveen Raj
Title: Conquering Obesity, Conquering Mountains
ISBN: 978-1-77371-614-5
Category: HEALTH & FITNESS/Diet & Nutrition/Weight Loss
Publisher: Mastery Books
Room 803, Tung Hip Commercial Building, 248 Des Voeux Road Central, Sheung Wan, Hong Kong

....

TABLE OF CONTENTS

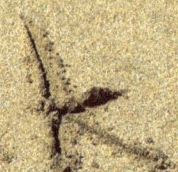

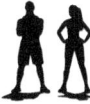

ACKNOWLEDGEMENT

This book, *Conquering Obesity, Conquering Mountains*, was written by authors Bruce Fam, Coach Aizat, and Praveen Raj (Sam) with consistent hard work and effort, so that individuals who are obese or overweight can find their path to conquering their own mountain of obesity and living a healthy life. However, the authors could not have achieved this feat without the help and support of many incredible individuals who worked tirelessly or supported us behind the scenes.

We would like to extend our deepest gratitude and thanks to:

- Our families and spouses for their patience and understanding while we dedicated time to writing this book.

- Gerry Robert and his wonderful team members, including Louie Acosta, Leesa Landry, and Anna Dowe, for providing professional guidance and support in publishing this book.

- Vince Tan and World MasterClass for providing invaluable knowledge, advice, and confidence during Bruce's initial journey in starting his business, WBF Healthy Living Sdn. Bhd.

ACKNOWLEDGEMENT

- The Board of Directors, management, and colleagues of the multinational companies where Bruce worked for a total of 39 years:

  o Texas Instruments Malaysia Sdn. Bhd. (1983–1992) as Facilities Maintenance Supervisor & Health, Safety, and Environmental (HSE) Engineer.

  o LOTTE Chemical Titan (M) Sdn. Bhd. (1992–2022) as Safety & Health Officer (SHO), HSE Engineer, Manager, and Director of Safety and Environment.

Bruce's extensive technical knowledge, experience, and training in health and safety, gained while working in these esteemed companies, contributed greatly to the writing of this book. He wishes to acknowledge their invaluable indirect contributions.

Lastly, we would like to thank all those who have directly or indirectly contributed to the success of this book.

FOREWORD BY GERRY ROBERT

I n a world dominated by quick fixes and fleeting trends, it is rare to find a book that approaches the challenge of weight loss with the depth, care, and practicality found in *Conquering Obesity, Conquering Mountains: 6 Steps to Fail-Proof, Sustainable Weight Loss and a Healthy Lifestyle Through a Holistic System*. This is more than just a guide to shedding pounds; it's a complete roadmap to transforming your health, your mindset, and ultimately your life.

I know firsthand the struggles that come with weight loss. Like many, I have faced challenges with my own weight over the years and experienced the physical and emotional toll it can take. I also understand the incredible commitment it requires to achieve lasting change. That's why this book resonates so deeply with me—it not only acknowledges these challenges but provides a clear, actionable system for overcoming them.

What sets this book apart is its holistic approach. It doesn't rely on gimmicks or promise overnight success. Instead, it empowers you with a proven six-step framework designed to address the root causes of weight gain, while offering practical tools for sustainable improvement. From understanding your priorities and aligning your mind and body to using strategies like the Plan-Do-Check-Act cycle and SWOT analysis, this book gives you the resources to achieve real, lasting results.

I admire the authors' ability to address the unique struggles of weight loss while focusing on the big picture: building a healthier, happier life. The emphasis here isn't just on losing the pounds but on reclaiming control over your choices, overcoming setbacks, and fostering continuous growth.

If you're reading this, you've already taken an important step toward conquering not just obesity but the mountains that may feel insurmountable in your life. Whether you're just beginning your journey or seeking a new way forward, the strategies in these pages will guide you with clarity, compassion, and purpose.

Take it from someone who has walked a similar path—this process works. It requires effort, resilience, and patience, but the rewards are life-changing. With this book, you'll not only gain the tools to transform your body but also the mindset to conquer challenges and create the life you truly deserve.

To your health and success,
Gerry Robert
Speaker and international bestselling author of *The Millionaire Mindset*, *Multiply Your Business* and *Publish a Book and Grow Rich*

PREFACE

Bruce Fam's Story on Conquering Obesity and Climbing Life's Mountains

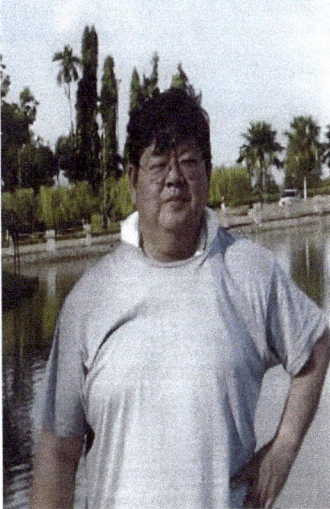

2017
114kg

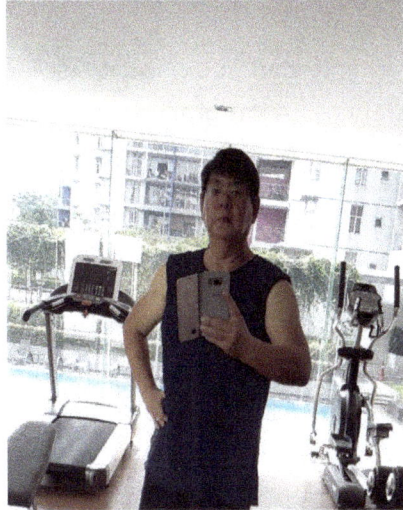

2021
86kg

Here is my journey, started in 2017 and having conquered mountains of obesity in 2021, without any medication or shortcuts, all with the power of will power.

My Personal Journey to Health and a 28 kg Weight Loss

For over 30 years, I dedicated my energy to a demanding career as a Safety and Health Officer, Engineer, and Director of Occupational Health, Safety, and Environment at one of Southeast Asia's largest petrochemical complexes. It was a high-pressure, high-stakes environment that left little time for anything else. Yet, behind my professional achievements, I carried a personal struggle that often left me feeling helpless and defeated—my battle with obesity.

Before I share my story, let me ask you a life-changing question: Which path will you choose to live your life?

- A healthy, safe, and successful career or business?

- A successful career or business at the cost of poor health and a weak safety culture?

The first path belongs to someone who prioritizes health and safety as an integral part of their life. The second prioritizes wealth, career, or business above all else.

If you choose the first path, keep reading—this is exactly what my story and *Conquering Obesity, Conquering Mountains* is all about.

Year after year, my health was a growing concern. Annual medical checkups showed troubling results: fatty liver, borderline cholesterol levels, and all the warning signs of a body under strain. I lived with the constant fear that my health would collapse, yet I felt trapped in my circumstances. Despite trying numerous diets and approaches, I couldn't lose weight and keep it off. The sense of hopelessness was overwhelming.

There were moments when I questioned everything. I often thought about quitting my job, convinced that my health, and ultimately my life, wasn't worth the paycheck and benefits. I even joked with my colleagues that I might be healthier working as a fisherman, staying active in the sun, surrounded by the beauty of the seaside. Of course, the reality was that I couldn't afford such a lifestyle due to mortgages, high living expenses, and financial obligations tied to my demanding career.

As the years passed, I couldn't escape the emotional toll obesity was taking on me. I felt angry, frustrated, and desperate. How could someone like me—educated, informed, and financially secure—not figure out how to lose weight? I couldn't help but think, "If I'm struggling this much, what about those who don't have the same resources?"

The Turning Point

In 2017, everything changed. I was in my late fifties, weighed 114 kilograms, and was at a critical juncture in my life. My lifestyle was unhealthy by every measure:

- I smoked until my mid-thirties.

- I drank occasionally.

- I was a heavy eater, a fast eater, and loved sugary foods.

- I lived a sedentary lifestyle and never exercised.

- I had a 24/7 job that left little time for self-care.

One day, I decided enough was enough. I resolved to take charge of my health with an ambitious goal: to lose weight and achieve a six-pack body within five years—or risk running out of time to turn my life around. This was my "Do or Die" moment, and I committed fully to the journey ahead to conquering my Obesity, conquering Mountains.

> *"Every mountain top is within reach if you just keep climbing."*
>
> **— Barry Finlay**,
> Kilimanjaro and Beyond

The Journey

The road was anything but easy. Changing lifelong habits required discipline and resilience. I had to fight against food cravings, temptations, the pull of old routines, and the inevitable setbacks that come with such a challenging goal. But I refused to give up.

I made weight loss an integral part of my life's priorities, alongside health and safety, wealth creation, a successful career and business, family and friends, spirituality, and other important areas of my life. I also fully embraced the fact that my health and safety must always come first. After all, if I were unhealthy or sick, all the wealth, success, and achievements in the world would mean nothing, I wouldn't live long or well enough to enjoy them.

Throughout my 30 years as a Health and Safety Professional, my team and I conducted hundreds of Health, Safety, and Environment (HSE) training sessions and meetings. Over the years, I asked thousands of people how they viewed the importance of HSE practices in their workplace. Almost all would confidently declare, *"HSE is our No. 1 priority!"*

Unfortunately, for many, these words were just *lip service*. In reality, they didn't truly prioritize safety, at least, not until a serious accident, injury, or death occurred. By then, it was too late. The same pattern applies to health. Many people place wealth, career, business, and social life above their well-being—until they experience a health scare or illness that forces them to reevaluate their priorities.

Thankfully, in my late fifties, I recognized this mistake before it was too late. I took action and conquered my obesity using a system now known as *The 6 Steps to Fail-Proof, Sustainable Weight Loss and a Healthy Lifestyle Through a Holistic System.*

Over time, I began to see progress. I focused on healthier eating, stayed active, and learned to listen to my body. Slowly but surely, I started to transform, not just physically, but mentally and emotionally as well.

Major Challenges, Obstacles and Disruptions Encountered and Ways to Overcome

Throughout my journey, I faced numerous unplanned challenges, obstacles, and disruptions in various roles: as a family head, a working professional, and an active member of society. Even something as routine as festive seasons (Christmas, Hari Raya Puasa, Deepavali, Chinese New Year), public holidays, and vacations could easily disrupt my nutrition plan, exercise routine, monitoring programs, and mindset. These disruptions threatened to undo weeks or months of progress.

Over time, I learned the importance of pre-planning contingency actions to minimize setbacks. For example, when traveling for a family vacation, I ensured the hotel had a swimming pool or gym so I could maintain my exercise routine. I also consciously planned to avoid overeating, especially at buffets. While this may seem trivial, managing these events was crucial in maintaining my hard-earned progress.

One of the biggest realizations in my journey was that weight gain happens quickly, but burning excess calories is much harder. Consider this: eating two Big Mac burgers adds approximately 1,054 calories, while an 85 kg person swimming casually for an hour burns only about 587 calories. That's a 467-calorie surplus, which gets stored as fat. This simple fact motivated me to adopt a powerful habit: before eating or drinking anything, I would calculate the equivalent physical effort needed to burn those calories. If the effort was too strenuous, I would adjust my portions or opt for lower-calorie alternatives.

As the Director of Safety and Environment in a petrochemical complex, I faced another significant challenge—an unpredictable and demanding work schedule. Given the hazardous nature of the materials and chemicals in our plants, health, safety, and environmental (HSE) considerations were always the top priority. Neglecting them could lead to fires, explosions, toxic material releases, severe injuries, or even fatalities.

While my official working hours were Monday to Friday, 8:30 AM – 5:30 PM, the reality was vastly different. Safety, environmental, and regulatory issues required my team and me to be available 24/7, year-round. Many nights, I had to rush back to the plant to handle emergencies, accidents, or shutdowns. During major plant maintenance shutdowns (turnarounds), I often spent 12+ hours per day on-site for 1-2 months straight.

With such an unpredictable schedule, planning workouts was extremely difficult. To overcome this, I took a practical approach:

- I kept my gym gear and Personal Protective Equipment (PPE) in my car so I could work out and still respond to emergencies immediately if needed.

- I arrived at work early (7:45 AM) to walk or bike around the plant for an hour while conducting daily safety inspections. With our facility spanning 200 acres, including high platforms and towers, this provided an excellent opportunity for physical activity.

- I took the stairs instead of the elevator whenever possible.

- I walked or biked to nearby stores or restaurants instead of driving.

By integrating physical activity into my daily responsibilities, I turned a potential time constraint into a win-win situation—improving my health while fulfilling my job requirements.

Another unavoidable disruption was illness and injury. Occasional flu, fever, colds, or muscle strains could temporarily halt my exercise routine. These setbacks were frustrating, as they often disrupted my calorie deficit. However, I learned to adapt and manage my nutrition by:

- Eating lighter, lower-calorie foods like oats, porridge, and soups.

- Staying hydrated and getting plenty of rest.

- Doing light walking instead of high-intensity workouts until I fully recovered.

During the COVID-19 pandemic, when gyms were closed, I purchased dumbbells to continue strength training at home, ensuring I didn't lose progress.

Through experience, I realized that these "pit stops"—times of rest, recovery, and self-evaluation—were just as important as periods of intense effort. Instead of viewing setbacks as failures, I saw them as opportunities to rejuvenate, manage stress, and maintain my achievements before pushing forward again.

> *"You have to conquer every obstacle, before you can reach the top of the mountain."*
>
> **— Lailah Gifty Akita**,
> Pearls of Wisdom

Taking Care of Ailing Parents (2006-2014)

One of the most challenging periods in my life was caring for my aging parents, who had lived independently in a small town in Johor, Malaysia. My mother had always been exceptionally healthy and active. Even in her mid-seventies, she maintained her home meticulously, practiced Tai Chi, and took daily walks. She took pride in rarely needing medical attention for common ailments like colds and fevers.

However, in 2006, everything changed. Without any prior warning, she suddenly fainted and had to be rushed to the hospital. After several tests, she was diagnosed with stage 2/3 stomach cancer. Over the next three years, until her passing in 2009, my family and I devoted almost all our free time to her care: coordinating her surgery, follow-up treatments, and daily needs. During this period, my father also began exhibiting signs of dementia, which progressively worsened.

After my mother's passing, the responsibility of caring for my father became even more demanding. His condition required constant attention, and balancing this alongside a full-time job was incredibly challenging. Until his passing in 2014, most of my free time was spent ensuring his well-being, making those years some of the most exhausting and emotionally draining of my life.

During this time, prioritizing my own health became nearly impossible. Exercise took a backseat, and I had little to no time to monitor my diet. As a result, my weight increased significantly. This situation is something many caregivers, especially working parents with young children, can relate to. The responsibility of caring for loved ones can be all-consuming, leaving little room for self-care.

In hindsight, knowing what I do now about health and wellness, I recognize that there were strategies I could have implemented to maintain my well-being even under these circumstances.

Here are some key approaches that could have helped:

1. **Maintaining a Caloric Deficit**

   A calorie deficit of 3,500 calories per week (or 500 calories per day) is essential for losing 0.45 kg (1 lb) of fat per week. Some ways to achieve this include:

   - Tracking caloric intake: Using apps or a food diary to monitor daily food consumption.

   - Eating nutrient-dense foods: Prioritizing fruits, vegetables, whole grains, lean proteins, and healthy fats to stay full while consuming fewer calories.

   - Controlling portion sizes: Using smaller plates and being mindful of serving sizes.

   - Staying hydrated: Drinking plenty of water to avoid mistaking thirst for hunger.

   - Consistency: Maintaining caloric goals daily to sustain progress.

   - Incorporating movement into daily life:

     o Using a treadmill or dumbbells at home.

     o Parking further from the office to increase daily steps.

     o Taking the stairs instead of the elevator.

     o Walking around the house or workplace during breaks.

- Adjusting when necessary: If weight loss stagnates, reassessing food intake and activity levels to make necessary modifications.

2. **Managing Mind-Body Balance**

Caring for ailing parents is both physically and emotionally draining. Prioritizing mental well-being is crucial:

- Practicing meditation, yoga, or spiritual prayers to reduce stress.

- Establishing a proper sleep routine for rest and recovery.

- Engaging in brisk walking or light exercise to boost mood and energy levels.

3. **Implementing a Plan-Do-Check-Act (PDCA) Cycle**

A structured approach to health and weight management can be beneficial even during challenging times:

- Plan: Set a three-month goal for weight management.

- Do: List the necessary activities to achieve the goal.

- Check: Monitor progress and track results.

- Act: Perform a SWOT analysis (Strengths, Weaknesses, Opportunities, Threats) to refine strategies for the next cycle.

4. **Seeking Support**

Caregiving can be overwhelming, and seeking help is essential:

- Reaching out to friends, colleagues, and relatives for assistance.

- Exploring support from welfare institutions or community services when needed.

Caring for loved ones is a profound responsibility, but it should not come at the expense of one's own health. With careful planning, small daily adjustments, and a strong support system, it is possible to balance caregiving while maintaining personal well-being.

Overcoming Hunger Pangs, Exhaustion and Weight Loss Plateaus

Throughout my journey, one of the most difficult challenges I faced was the psychological and mental strain caused by hunger pangs. These often occurred when I ate smaller portions at lunch or dinner or increased my exercise. At times, I experienced stomach growling, low energy, and even fainting spells due to prolonged hunger. Instead of secretly consuming unhealthy, high-calorie snacks or junk food, which would undermine my calorie deficit, I found that low-calorie protein bars or meal replacement options, such as nutritious soy protein shakes, provided a good temporary solution. A 25-gram soy protein shake mixed with water contains only 99 calories, making it an effective option. However, maintaining this approach long-term can be expensive. As a compromise, I used these meal replacements strategically, especially during festive seasons when my exercise routine was less consistent. A more affordable alternative was low-calorie oat bars, which are both healthy and cost-effective. I made it a rule to avoid salty, carbohydrate-heavy snacks like potato chips or fries, as they could easily derail my progress.

Another effective strategy for managing hunger pangs was consuming low-calorie, less-sweet fruits like apples, pears, and pineapples, as well as vegetables like cucumbers. Additionally, drinking plenty of water helped curb cravings, as thirst is often mistaken for hunger.

Exhaustion and weight loss plateaus can be particularly demotivating if we don't understand the complexities of the weight loss process. As I mentioned earlier, conquering obesity is like conquering a mountain—it requires persistence, patience, adaptability, and a positive attitude. Throughout my journey, I encountered physical, mental, and emotional fatigue, all of which contributed to exhaustion. Addressing these challenges was crucial to maintaining progress.

Physical fatigue is a natural response when engaging in physical activity or following a new diet. Our bodies undergo significant changes, including increased energy expenditure, muscle soreness, and an overall adjustment period. While physical fatigue is normal, if not managed properly, it can become a barrier to achieving weight loss goals.

Beyond physical exhaustion, mental fatigue also plays a major role in weight loss struggles. As busy professionals, we juggle numerous responsibilities, and the constant mental strain can leave us feeling drained and unmotivated. Negative thoughts, self-doubt, and lack of mental clarity can make it difficult to stay on track. Furthermore, emotional fatigue, triggered by stress, emotional eating, and coping mechanisms, can take a toll on overall well-being. The ups and downs of weight loss often bring emotional roller coasters, leading to moments of discouragement and exhaustion. Recognizing these emotional triggers is essential for developing strategies to overcome them.

To combat exhaustion, I adopted a holistic approach that incorporated both physical and mental well-being. One of the most crucial aspects of overcoming exhaustion was cultivating a positive and resilient mindset. It's easy to get discouraged when faced with setbacks or plateaus. However, maintaining a positive outlook and believing in my ability to succeed made all the difference. Instead of focusing on what went wrong, I chose to celebrate small victories and acknowledge my progress. This mindset shift, one of resilience and perseverance, helped me push through difficult moments and stay committed to my journey.

Building a strong support system also proved invaluable. Surrounding myself with individuals who supported my weight loss goals, such as a gym trainer, nutritionist, or positive-minded colleagues, provided motivation and encouragement. Support could come from friends, family, or even online communities on platforms like Facebook, YouTube, or LinkedIn. However, I remained cautious, as misinformation is rampant online and can easily mislead, demotivate, or derail progress. Engaging with a trustworthy support network helped me stay accountable and inspired.

Self-care was another critical factor in overcoming exhaustion. Many professionals neglect their well-being in pursuit of career success, but taking care of oneself physically, mentally, and emotionally is essential for sustainable weight loss. I incorporated activities that brought me joy and helped me recharge, whether it was a relaxing bath, yoga, reading, or spending quality time with loved ones. Prioritizing self-care allowed me to replenish my energy and find balance in my life.

Proper nutrition and hydration were also key in maintaining energy levels. I ensured that my diet was well-balanced, rich in whole foods, lean proteins, complex carbohydrates, and healthy fats. These nutrient-dense choices provided sustained energy throughout the day. Hydration was equally important, as even mild dehydration could contribute to fatigue. I made it a habit to drink plenty of water and limit my intake of sugary and caffeinated beverages.

Additionally, incorporating regular movement into my daily routine helped combat both physical and mental exhaustion. Exercise not only aids in weight loss but also releases endorphins, which boost mood and energy levels. I found activities I enjoyed, such as walking, fitness classes, and team sports, which made it easier to stay consistent. By making exercise a non-negotiable part of my lifestyle, I was able to maintain motivation and avoid burnout.

As I have shared, the journey to conquering obesity is not easy. The road to weight loss is filled with challenges: time constraints, demanding jobs, external and internal obstacles, festive seasons, vacations, hunger pangs, mental and physical exhaustion, and frustrating plateaus. However, through my personal experience, I developed the 6 *Steps to Fail-Proof, Sustainable Weight Loss and a Healthy Lifestyle Through a Holistic System*. This system provided a structured path for me to overcome obesity, and I am confident that it can guide others as well. Today, I can say with certainty that I have the tools to lose weight and maintain it for life, as long as I follow the six steps outlined in this book. As I emphasized earlier, success requires patience, consistency, and allowing the body sufficient time to respond in a healthy manner.

The Result: A New Me

By 2021, I had reduced my weight from 114 kg to a lean 86 kg, losing a total of 28 kilograms. It wasn't just about the weight loss; it was about the freedom and vitality I gained in the process.

- I learned to control my food cravings.

- My energy levels returned, and I felt alive in a way I hadn't in decades.

- I became more active, more focused, and more present in my life.

While I didn't quite achieve the six-pack body I had envisioned, I succeeded in reclaiming my health and conquering the mountain of obesity that had weighed me down for so long.

"There's no glory in climbing a mountain if all you want to do is to get to the top. It's experiencing the climb itself—in all its moments of revelation, heartbreak, and fatigue—that has to be the goal."

—Karyn Kusama

Why I Developed the 6 Steps to Fail-Proof, Sustainable Weight Loss and a Healthy Lifestyle Through a Holistic System

During my weight loss journey, as I started seeing tangible results—my body weight dropping from 114 kg and my pants size reducing from 42 inches to 40 inches—people at my workplace and friends began to notice the changes. Many of them, struggling with similar weight issues, asked about my weight loss method and my "secret." While I tried to explain, I found it difficult because there were so many aspects to cover, and repeating the details became tiring. To provide a more comprehensive response, I decided to compile my experiences, conduct proper research, and develop a structured system. This led to the creation of the 6 Steps Holistic System.

During this time, I was fortunate to meet Praveen Raj (Sam), who, through our shared interest in overcoming life challenges and our business relationship, agreed to co-author this book and partner in my business. Later, we also had the privilege of connecting with Coach Aizat, who holds a BSc in Health Science (Nutrition) and is a National Academy of Sports Medicine (NASM) Performance Enhancement Specialist. Coach Aizat joined us as both a co-author of this book and a business partner.

Both Praveen Raj (Sam) and Coach Aizat have made significant contributions to enhancing the *6 Steps to Fail-Proof, Sustainable Weight Loss and a Healthy Lifestyle Through a Holistic System*. As the authors of *Conquering Obesity, Conquering Mountains*, we have poured our best efforts into writing this book, with the hope that it will help millions of obese and overweight individuals worldwide conquer their obesity, overcome their personal mountains, and live a healthier life.

Why I'm Sharing My Story

One of the most heartbreaking aspects of my journey in conquering extreme obesity and reclaiming my health in my late fifties is my inability to share my experience and knowledge with many of my friends who suffered from serious illnesses such as diabetes and heart disease due to obesity/being overweight. Their suffering, and ultimately their untimely deaths, could have been prevented, in my view, through our *6 Steps to Achieve Fail-Proof, Sustainable Weight Loss and a Healthy Lifestyle Through a Systematic and Holistic Approach.*

Even more concerning, today we see hundreds of millions of obese/ overweight individuals, both young and old, who remain unaware of the severe risks and hidden dangers of obesity/overweight. Their lack of urgency may stem from years of frustration and disappointment after repeated failed attempts to lose weight and conquer their obesity. In the next section, we will explore the emotional stress and psychological stages that an obese person experiences during the challenging journey of weight loss and adopting a healthy lifestyle.

Looking back, I know how isolating and overwhelming the weight loss journey can feel. It's not just about eating less or moving more; it's about navigating the physical, mental, and emotional challenges that come with such a significant transformation.

The purpose of this book is to share and educate people on how to overcome their overweight or obesity challenges through a holistic, fail-proof system. This system, called the *6 Steps to Fail-Proof, Sustainable Weight Loss and a Healthy Lifestyle Through a Holistic System*, empowers individuals to gain clarity and a full understanding of the challenges they will face on the journey. More importantly, it emphasizes that consistent efforts are required to conquer obesity and achieve sustainable, healthy living.

The analogy of Conquering Mountains is central to this book because the journey to lose weight is much like scaling multiple mountains of physical obstacles, mental barriers, emotional struggles, and lifestyle changes. It requires preparation, persistence, and the ability to push through these challenges, one at a time. Each step forward might feel slow and grueling at times, but with consistent effort and determination, the summits are within reach.

I've been where you are, and I understand the struggles you're facing. This book is my way of showing you that with the right mindset, tools, and support, you can conquer your own mountains and live a healthy, safe, vibrant, and empowered life.

"The hardest mountain to climb is the one within."

—J. Lynn

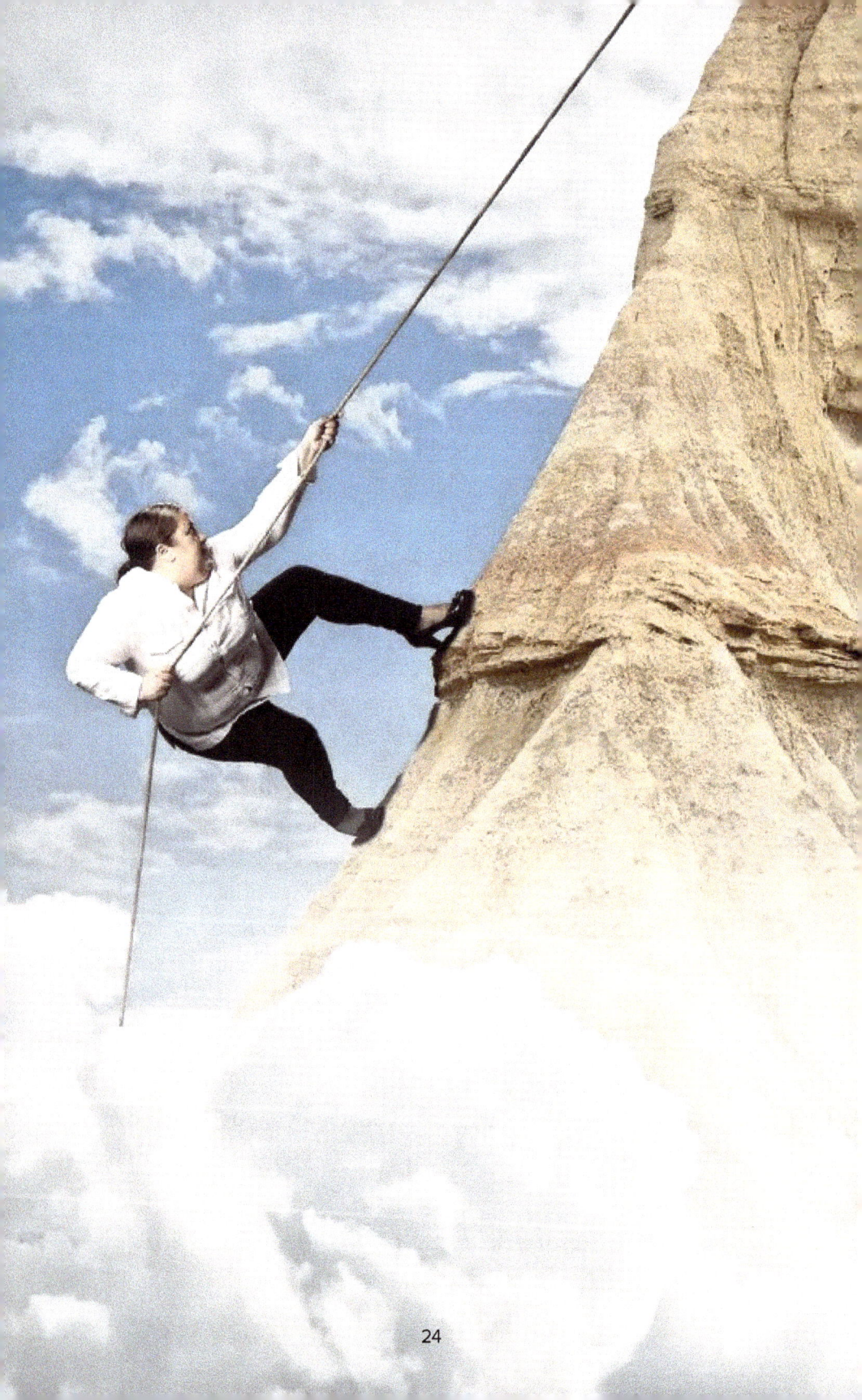

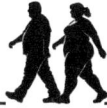

INTRODUCTION

Welcome to *Conquering Obesity, Conquering Mountains: 6 Steps to Fail-Proof, Sustainable Weight Loss and a Healthy Lifestyle Through a Holistic System*. This book is not just about conquering obesity by losing weight; it's about transforming your life by treating the weight loss journey as an integral part of your overall success. Achieving good health and well-being impacts every aspect of life, including personal safety, financial stability, career and business success, relationships with family and friends, spirituality, and more. The 6 Steps System integrates the 8 essential elements of healthy living, along with a positive mental attitude, success principles, life priorities, and the alignment of mind, body, and consciousness into a holistic approach to lasting transformation.It is the culmination of years of experience, personal growth, and a deep understanding of what it truly takes mentally and physically to conquer obesity and live a healthy & safe, balanced successful life. Whether you are just beginning your weight loss journey or have struggled with maintaining a healthy lifestyle in the past, this book is here to guide you through every step of the process.

What Makes This Book's 6-Step System for Fail-Proof, Sustainable Weight Loss and a Healthy Lifestyle Unique?

The weight loss industry is a massive global business, offering countless methods such as special diets like Keto, Intermittent Fasting, and the Mediterranean Diet, as well as low-carb meal replacements, weight loss drugs, and various non-surgical treatments, including CoolSculpting, ultrasound or radiofrequency treatments, electrical muscle stimulation, and body contouring services. Surgical procedures and dietary supplements are also widely promoted, each catering to different individual needs and preferences. These commercialized solutions often come at a high cost, making them inaccessible to many. With so many weight loss methods available, one might wonder why over 800 million people worldwide remain obese, with numbers continuing to rise, according to the World Health Organization (WHO).

This ongoing issue highlights a fundamental problem—these weight loss methods are not effectively helping the majority of the global obese population achieve sustained weight loss. Several key reasons contribute to this failure.

- Results are not guaranteed: Non-surgical options often produce inconsistent results and are generally less effective than a long-term commitment to proper nutrition, regular physical exercise, daily healthy activities, appropriate food supplements, continuous monitoring, and a positive mental attitude.

- Health risks: Any medical procedure carries potential risks, including complications and side effects. It is essential to consult a qualified healthcare professional before undergoing any treatment.

- Not a substitute for healthy habits: Liposuction and similar treatments do not replace the long-term benefits of a balanced diet and regular physical activity. Sustainable weight loss requires a commitment to healthy living.

- Treatments are costly: Many commercial weight loss solutions, including medical procedures and specialized diets, can be expensive and may not be financially sustainable for long-term use.

In summary, while shortcuts may seem appealing, real, sustainable results come from a commitment to healthy living. This book introduces the *6 Steps to Fail-Proof, Sustainable Weight Loss and a Healthy Lifestyle Through a Holistic System*, which focuses on natural, step-by-step weight loss. This approach emphasizes lifestyle changes, eliminating poor eating habits, increasing physical activity, and encouraging continuous improvement day after day, week after week, month after month, and year after year, throughout one's lifetime.

What makes this system so unique and special? A system is defined as "a set of things working together as parts of a mechanism or an interconnecting network; a complex whole." Think of the traffic system, where traffic lights help vehicles move orderly at busy junctions. The simple procedure of "Red is for Stop," "Yellow is to Slow down," and "Green is to Move" ensures smooth and safe traffic flow. Imagine a world without traffic lights—driving at junctions would be chaotic.

Similarly, our 6-STEP System allows someone who is obese to set a goal of losing a specific amount of body weight, take actions such as reducing sugar and carbohydrates, and monitor progress over the next 3 months. After 3 months, the individual can perform a simple

Strengths-Weaknesses-Opportunities-Threats (SWOT) review to evaluate what worked well, what didn't, the opportunities that arose, and the challenges faced during the journey. By actively engaging in this 3-month cycle and reflecting on the progress, the person will significantly reduce the fear of failure, lack of confidence, and insecurity. The system requires repeating this 3-month journey a second time, but with a better understanding, clearer expectations, and increased vigor, as the person becomes more confident and knowledgeable about the weight loss process. This iterative cycle continues, fostering a healthier lifestyle, improved eating habits, and greater physical activity, making weight loss sustainable over the long term.

Additionally, this system allows the individual to chart a path that aligns with their unique temperament, lifestyle, and special circumstances. It is like creating a personalized journey to conquer obesity and face the challenges of life, much like summiting a mountain.

"When you stand at the bottom of the mountain and look up at the mountaintop, the path looks hard and stony, and the top is obscured by clouds. But when you reach the top and you look down, you realize that there are a thousand paths that could have brought you to that place."

— Roz Savage,
Rowing the Atlantic: Lessons Learned on the Open Ocean

The weight loss journey is highly personal and varies from person to person. As Coach Aizat frequently advises his clients, there is no one-size-fits-all "best" diet. Each individual's optimal dietary approach is unique to their lifestyle and needs. Blindly following someone else's diet simply because it worked for them can lead to a frustrating cycle of yo-yo dieting. Similarly, when it comes to physical exercise and daily activities, each person should choose the sports and activities that suit their preferences and needs, as everyone is different. The uniqueness of our system lies in in the following key aspects:

- **Empowering individuals with proper knowledge:** In Chapter 4, we provide an understanding of the 8 Essential Elements of Healthy Living. Without a clear understanding of these elements, achieving sustainable weight loss becomes nearly impossible. Without proper knowledge, it is like being led around with a leash on your neck, especially given the vast amount of misinformation circulating in the media. It can be disheartening and confusing to navigate the weight loss journey due to half-truths, exaggerated claims, self-interests, lies, or fake news propagated by some sources.

- **Incorporating weight loss into life priorities and goals:** Weight loss should be viewed as an integral part of one's life goals, such as health and safety, wealth creation, career success, and relationships with family and friends. However, it is essential to recognize that health and safety must always be the top priority. Without good health, all the wealth, career achievements, and businesses mean little, as one will not be able to enjoy them if their health is compromised.

- **Incorporating continuous improvement methodologies:** The system integrates step-by-step methodologies like Plan-Do-Check-Act (PDCA) and Strength-Weaknesses-Opportunities-Threats (SWOT) to ensure continuous progress in the lifelong weight loss journey.

- **Taking action every 3 months with a SWOT review:** A simple SWOT review every 3 months helps reduce the fear of failure and insecurity, boosts confidence, and allows for adaptability and flexibility. This approach enables an individual to chart their own unique path to conquer obesity, just as one would conquer mountains.

Overview of the Book's Purpose

The goal isn't just to gain knowledge, but to put it into action. Nearly 90% of people give up after the first few weeks, which is why so many journeys end in failure.

The purpose of this book is to provide you with a holistic, sustainable system for weight loss that goes beyond quick fixes, fads, and temporary solutions. Through the 6-Step system that we developed from Bruce's own personal journey, you will learn not just how to lose weight, but how to keep it off long-term by creating lasting habits that support a healthy lifestyle. This system addresses the physical, mental, and emotional aspects of weight loss, providing a comprehensive approach that is tailored to your individual needs.

In these pages, you'll discover practical strategies for managing your time, stress, and mindset, all of which are integral to your success. You will also find tools to help you evaluate and refine your progress, ensuring that each step you take brings you closer to your goal. Most importantly, this book emphasizes that achieving a healthy weight is not just a destination—it's a lifelong journey of continuous improvement.

What to Expect and How to Use This Book Effectively

Each chapter of this book is designed to guide you through a specific aspect of your weight loss journey, from understanding the truth about obesity and why most people fail, to implementing the 6-Step cycle for continuous improvement in weight loss. As you read, you'll find a combination of theory, practical advice, and actionable steps that you can apply immediately to your life.

To get the most out of this book, I recommend the following approach:

1. **Read with Intention:** Take your time to absorb the information in each chapter. Don't rush through the content—focus on understanding the principles behind each step.

2. **Apply What You Learn:** As you read, try to implement the techniques and strategies outlined in each chapter. Each step builds on the previous one, so it's essential to apply the concepts as you go.

3. **Track Your Progress:** Use the tools and resources provided in the book, such as the tracking tools and healthy meal ideas in the Appendix, to monitor your progress and make adjustments as needed.

4. **Stay Committed:** Remember, weight loss is a journey. You will face challenges along the way, but with consistency, patience, and the right mindset, you will overcome them and achieve lasting success.

This book is designed to be a companion on your path to not only conquering obesity but also achieving a vibrant, healthy, and empowered life. I invite you to dive in, take action, and embrace the journey ahead. The mountains are waiting for you to conquer them. Let's get started!

The Weight Loss Challenge

Obesity is one of the greatest health challenges of our time, affecting millions of people across all demographics, professions, and walks of life. According to the World Health Organization's 2022 World Obesity Day report (revised February 2024), approximately 800 million people worldwide are obese. This includes 670 million adults and at least 120 million children and adolescents based on 2016 data—and this number continues to rise. Obesity is a major contributor to a range of non-communicable diseases (NCDs), including type 2 diabetes, cardiovascular disease, hypertension, stroke, various forms of cancer, and mental health issues.

Why is obesity so widespread today? Let me tell you something important: it's not your fault. The odds are stacked against you from the start. Everywhere you turn, you're surrounded by unhealthy fast food options, bright signs, and enticing smells designed to lure you in. Walk into a supermarket, and the shelves are lined with highly processed, sugar-laden products, carefully placed to catch your eye.

But why does it have to be this way? It all boils down to the simple goals of the food industry:

1. Cut costs.

2. Create repeat customers.

3. Increase profits.

To achieve these goals, companies rely on a dangerous combination—longer shelf life, addictive flavors, and larger portion sizes. They've mastered the science of keeping food cheap, delicious, and nearly irresistible. Every bite is carefully engineered to hit the "bliss point" in your brain, releasing a flood of dopamine that makes you crave more.

Think about it: how often have you opened a bag of chips, promising yourself just a few, only to find the bag empty before you know it? It's not a lack of willpower—it's by design. And behind that design is an industry more focused on their bottom line than your well-being.

The strategy is simple: make products as addictive as possible to drive repeat purchases and increase profits. But what's the real cost? Our health, our confidence, and our future.

So, how do we live healthy lives in a world that preys on our vulnerabilities? It starts with awareness and, most importantly, taking back control. This is where your mind becomes your greatest ally. Learning to resist these subtle traps and build sustainable habits isn't easy, but it's the key to living above the noise.

In the face of a system designed to profit from our weaknesses, your greatest power is to understand, adapt, and rise stronger. Let's explore how you can break free from these patterns and thrive, not just survive, in a world full of hidden temptations.

The COVID-19 pandemic further highlighted the risks associated with obesity, with individuals affected being three times more likely to be hospitalized. This begs the question: *Why is obesity such a massive global issue, and why haven't advancements in technology and artificial intelligence (AI) provided a solution to this life-threatening epidemic?*

As someone who has personally experienced the struggles of obesity throughout most of my adult life, I can attest to the physical, mental, and emotional toll it takes. I was fortunate to overcome this condition in my late fifties, losing 28 kilograms just in time to reclaim my health. In this book, I share my story, not just to inspire but to show that overcoming obesity is possible—even in the face of overwhelming odds.

Interestingly, obesity is not confined to those with limited resources or knowledge. Even some of the world's wealthiest individuals, influential leaders, and highly educated professionals—Emperors, Presidents, Prime Ministers, billionaires, doctors, lawyers, engineers—suffer from obesity. Despite their access to resources, many still struggle to address this condition.

To make matters worse, statistics show that approximately 90% of people who lose a significant amount of weight regain it over time. Why is sustainable weight loss so challenging? The answer lies in the multifaceted and deeply complex nature of the problem. Some key factors include:

1. **Lifestyle Choices:** Unhealthy eating habits such as overeating, consuming sugary drinks, eating high-carb foods, and excessive alcohol consumption. Additionally, a sedentary lifestyle with minimal physical activity exacerbates the issue.

2. **Biological Challenges:** The body works against weight loss efforts by slowing metabolism during weight loss and releasing hormonal signals that increase hunger, creating a persistent inner voice chanting, "Eat, eat, eat."

3. **Psychological Struggles:** Mental stress, emotional changes due to food deprivation, and the psychological impact of altering one's lifestyle or eating habits can undermine progress.

4. **Environmental Factors:** Stressful workplaces, peer pressure, financial challenges, and social disruptions can make sustainable weight loss feel insurmountable.

5. **Insufficient Sleep:** A lack of quality sleep negatively impacts metabolism and overall health.

6. **Dehydration:** Drinking insufficient water hampers bodily functions and metabolism, making weight loss more difficult.

Diagram 1: **FACTORS AFFECTING WEIGHT LOSS PERFORMANCE**

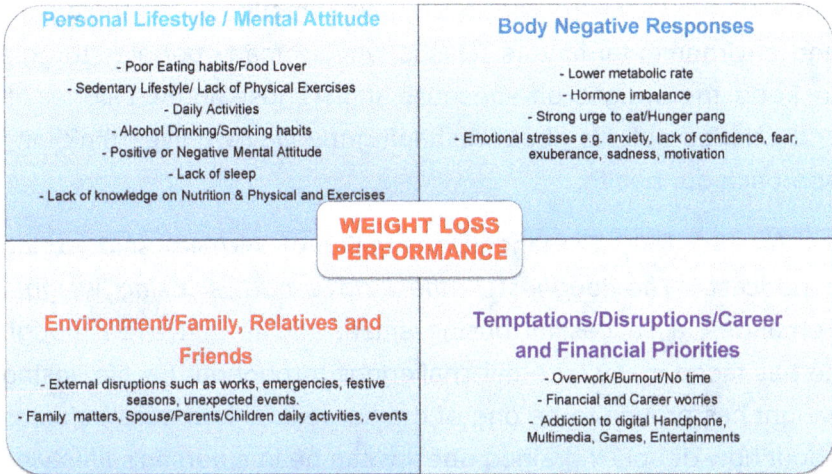

Personal Lifestyle / Mental Attitude	Body Negative Responses
- Poor Eating habits/Food Lover - Sedentary Lifestyle/ Lack of Physical Exercises - Daily Activities - Alcohol Drinking/Smoking habits - Positive or Negative Mental Attitude - Lack of sleep - Lack of knowledge on Nutrition & Physical and Exercises	- Lower metabolic rate - Hormone imbalance - Strong urge to eat/Hunger pang - Emotional stresses e.g. anxiety, lack of confidence, fear, exuberance, sadness, motivation
Environment/Family, Relatives and Friends	**Temptations/Disruptions/Career and Financial Priorities**
- External disruptions such as works, emergencies, festive seasons, unexpected events. - Family matters, Spouse/Parents/Children daily activities, events	- Overwork/Burnout/No time - Financial and Career worries - Addiction to digital Handphone, Multimedia, Games, Entertainments

WEIGHT LOSS PERFORMANCE

The Truth About Obesity

Obesity is often seen as a physical issue, but the truth is, it's far more complex. It's a multifaceted struggle that involves not just what we eat or how we move, but also how we think, feel, and live. It's a battle of willpower, of mindset, and of habits. This journey to better health and weight loss is not an easy one, and as many as 90% of people who successfully lose weight end up regaining it. Why is it that so many people fail to maintain their progress? What makes sustained success so elusive?

"Mountains are only a problem when they are bigger than you. You should develop yourself so much that you become bigger than the mountains you face."

—Idowu Koyenikan

The Real Struggle: A Multi-Dimensional Challenge

Losing weight isn't as simple as just eating less and exercising more. If it were that easy, the statistics would be far better. Obesity is a complex issue rooted in physical, emotional, psychological, and environmental factors. This is why so many people struggle to keep the weight off—because it isn't just about calories in and calories out. It's about reshaping the way we live, think, and approach our health.

As Tan Sri Tony Fernandes, the CEO of AirAsia, said during a podcast, *"The toughest battle I have had is losing weight."* Fernandes, a successful businessman, admits that even though he has faced many external challenges throughout his life, losing weight has proven to be one of the hardest. This speaks volumes about how deeply ingrained obesity can be in a person's lifestyle.

Dr. Katrina Ubell, MD, touches on another reality in her book, *How to Lose Weight for the Last Time*. She writes, *"We [doctors] are supposed to be experts on health. But here is the truth: Doctors learn very little about nutrition or how to maintain a healthy weight in medical school."* This statement highlights how widespread the knowledge gap about weight loss really is. Even healthcare professionals, who should be the experts in all things health-related, struggle to maintain healthy eating habits, which is reflected in the 63% of U.S. physicians being overweight or obese.

Diagram 2: EMOTIONAL STAGES** OF JOURNEY TO CONQUER OBESITY AND CONSEQUENCES OF FAILURE

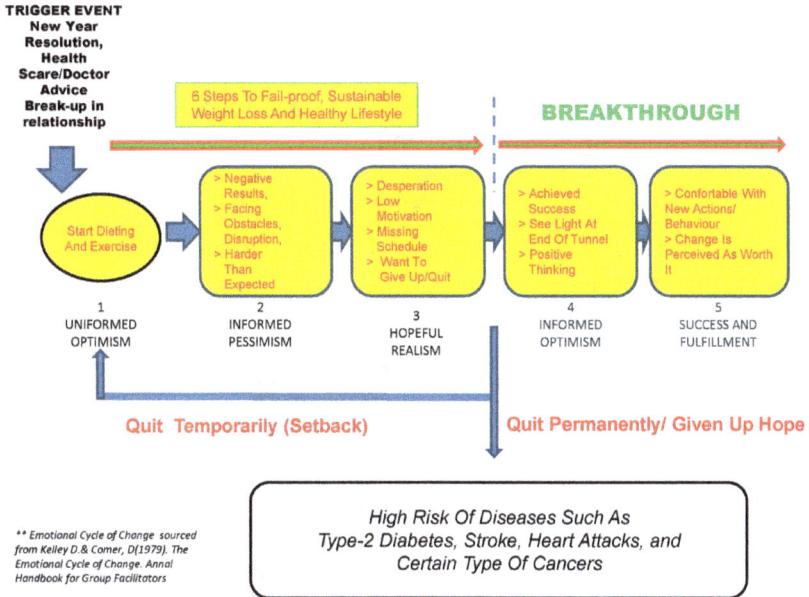

TRIGGER EVENT
New Year
Resolution,
Health
Scare/Doctor
Advice
Break-up in
relationship

6 Steps To Fail-proof, Sustainable Weight Loss And Healthy Lifestyle

BREAKTHROUGH

Start Dieting And Exercise

> Negative Results,
> Facing Obstacles, Disruption,
> Harder Than Expected

> Desperation
> Low Motivation
> Missing Schedule
> Want To Give Up/Quit

> Achieved Success
> See Light At End Of Tunnel
> Positive Thinking

> Comfortable With New Actions/ Behaviour
> Change Is Perceived As Worth It

1	2	3	4	5
UNIFORMED OPTIMISM	INFORMED PESSIMISM	HOPEFUL REALISM	INFORMED OPTIMISM	SUCCESS AND FULFILLMENT

Quit Temporarily (Setback)   Quit Permanently/ Given Up Hope

** Emotional Cycle of Change sourced from Kelley D.& Comer, D(1979). The Emotional Cycle of Change. Annal Handbook for Group Facilitators

High Risk Of Diseases Such As Type-2 Diabetes, Stroke, Heart Attacks, and Certain Type Of Cancers

Why 90% of People Fail to Keep the Weight Off

The journey to sustainable weight loss is difficult, and statistics show that 90% of those who lose weight will regain it within a few years. What are the reasons for this high failure rate? Why does it seem so hard to maintain weight loss? The answer lies in several common pitfalls that many of us fall into along the way. Before we dive into the pitfalls, let us consider the conflict of Pain vs Pleasure as part of our journey.

Pain vs. Pleasure: The Driving Forces Behind Every Action

At the core of every decision we make lies a simple equation: pain versus pleasure. These two forces drive our actions, often without us realizing it. If you break it down, every choice we make is an attempt to either avoid pain or seek pleasure.

Take a moment to reflect on this: Does exercising trigger pain or pleasure for you? Now compare that to the experience of eating a bag of chips. The answer is clear. Exercise is often associated with discomfort, such as muscle soreness, fatigue, and effort. On the other hand, chips offer instant gratification with a salty, crispy burst of flavor that feels rewarding in the moment.

Sure, you may feel guilty after polishing off the bag, but by then, it's too late. Your mind was locked on the immediate pleasure. Why? Because our brains are wired to prioritize short-term rewards over long-term benefits.

This brings us to the challenge of delayed gratification—the ability to resist immediate pleasure in exchange for a future reward. It's a skill we must train our minds to develop.

Reframing Exercise: From Pain to Purpose

To succeed, we must shift the way we view exercise and any habit-building activity. Instead of fixating on the immediate discomfort, we need to focus on the bigger picture—improved energy levels, a stronger and more resilient body, increased confidence, and long-term health and vitality.

But here's where it gets tricky: the outcome of exercise is often abstract and feels distant. You don't wake up leaner, stronger, or more energized after one workout. It takes weeks, sometimes months, for the results to become visible. This uncertainty makes it difficult for the mind to believe in the reward, especially when it craves tangible proof.

Why Junk Food Wins the Mental Battle

Compare that to eating a bag of chips. The pleasure is immediate and undeniable. The taste, the crunch, and the hit of dopamine in your brain all happen in seconds. The mind perceives this as a sure thing. The reward is real and instantaneous, while the potential downside such as guilt, bloating, or long-term health impacts feels distant or abstract.

This is why unhealthy habits are so easy to form but so difficult to break. They offer guaranteed pleasure without delay.

The Solution: Training the Mind for Long-Term Rewards

To live a healthier and more disciplined life, we must train our minds to shift focus from short-term gratification to long-term outcomes. Here is how you can start:

1. **Visualize the Future Outcome:** Create a mental image of what success looks like, such as stronger muscles, better sleep, and more energy. The clearer the vision, the more your mind starts to believe it.

2. **Celebrate Small Wins:** Reinforce the habit by rewarding yourself for small milestones, such as completing a week of workouts or saying no to junk food once a day. These small victories give the brain tangible evidence of progress.

3. **Make the Process Enjoyable:** Find ways to make the process itself pleasurable. Listen to music, work out with a friend, or track your progress to create a sense of accomplishment.

Connect Pain to Short-Term Pleasures

Another effective strategy is to associate pain with behaviors that derail your progress. Our minds naturally seek to avoid pain, so creating a mental link between short-term indulgence and discomfort can strengthen your resolve. For instance, you could set a rule for yourself: If I eat a bag of chips, I also need to eat a spoonful of something unappealing, like a can of cat food. While this example may sound extreme, the point is to condition your mind to link indulgence with an undesirable consequence. The stronger this association becomes, the higher the chance of resisting temptation.

However, this approach can be difficult to maintain on your own. Many people struggle to stay consistent without external accountability.

Leverage Accountability to Stay on Track

Having an accountability buddy who knows your goals and tracks your progress can make a significant difference. Knowing that someone else is observing your progress helps you stay focused and aware. When you feel tempted to give in, the thought of explaining the slip to your accountability partner can act as a deterrent.

If you do fall off track, your accountability partner can remind you of your commitment and encourage you to follow through on what you said you would do. This external reinforcement builds resilience, making you more likely to bounce back from setbacks and less likely to repeat the same mistakes.

By reinforcing the connection between setbacks and discomfort, while also creating a support system, you can train your mind to choose long-term rewards over fleeting pleasures. The journey may not be easy, but with the right mindset and support, it is absolutely achievable.

Mastering the Pain-Pleasure Balance

The key to mastering your habits is not about eliminating pleasure. It is about redefining it. Instead of associating pleasure solely with immediate gratification, train your mind to take pride in the strength you are building and the progress you are making.

When you can look past the short-term discomfort and embrace the long-term reward, you have unlocked one of the greatest strengths: the power to live intentionally rather than reactively.

In the battle between pain and pleasure, the winner is the one you feed. Which will you choose?

Now, let's dive into the common pitfalls why 90% of people fail to keep the weight off:

1. **The Wrong Mindset**

   The way we approach weight loss is often the first barrier. A negative mindset can sabotage even the most determined efforts. People tend to fall into a cycle of self-doubt, telling themselves things like, "This isn't working," "I've made mistakes, so I might as well quit," or "I'm not good enough to succeed at this." This kind of thinking can derail progress before it even starts.

   On the other hand, a positive, growth-oriented mindset can make all the difference. Instead of focusing on failure, those with a positive mindset see mistakes as opportunities to learn, grow, and improve. They embrace setbacks as part of the process, keep pushing forward, and refuse to give up. "I'll try a different approach," "Mistakes help me grow," and "I will keep trying until I succeed." These affirmations are the kind of positive thinking that propels individuals toward lasting success.

Cultural and social pressures, along with unrealistic standards set by the media, can create external stressors that challenge our ability to maintain focus on a healthy lifestyle. These pressures often lead to frustration, which can easily undermine progress, contributing to negative thinking and poor mindset.

2. **Unrealistic Expectations and Instant Gratification**

In today's world of instant gratification, it's easy to expect rapid results. Many people start their weight loss journey looking for a fast fix—something quick and easy. Crash diets and extreme workout programs promise rapid results, but the reality is that these approaches are rarely sustainable.

Social pressures, from social media influencers to celebrity endorsements, often exacerbate unrealistic expectations by promoting quick, superficial weight loss methods. These pressures make it harder to stick with realistic and sustainable changes.

The truth is, weight loss is a slow and steady process. Quick fixes might show short-term results, but they often lead to burnout and frustration. Delayed gratification, the ability to resist immediate rewards for long-term benefits, is crucial for lasting success. Sustainable weight loss is about making gradual, consistent changes that last for the long haul. Sacrificing today for a healthier tomorrow is the mindset that helps you scale the mountains of weight loss.

3. **Lack of Consistency**

One of the biggest challenges in maintaining weight loss is consistency. Many people go through cycles of strict dieting followed by periods of indulgence, only to see their hard-earned progress undone. Success requires building new habits and sticking to them consistently, even when motivation wanes.

Lack of monitoring, including tracking food intake and exercise, makes it difficult to stay on track. Without this consistent oversight, it becomes easier to lose focus, and small setbacks go unnoticed, turning into larger problems. Fluctuating exercise routines and inconsistent eating habits make it nearly impossible to achieve lasting results. Creating a sustainable routine—one that balances diet, exercise, and rest—is key to long-term success. When consistency becomes a habit, progress follows naturally.

Mindless eating—snacking while distracted, consuming larger portions than necessary, or eating out of boredom—also plays a role in undermining consistency. This habit can lead to overeating, making it difficult to sustain healthy habits.

4. **Poor Nutrition Knowledge**

There's no shortage of conflicting information when it comes to nutrition. Fad diets, misleading claims, and an overwhelming amount of dietary advice can leave people confused and unsure of what to eat. Without a solid understanding of what constitutes a balanced, nutritious diet, people often make poor food choices that derail their efforts.

Part of the problem is that many people don't truly understand nutrition or how to create a diet that supports weight loss. Mindless eating, poor planning, and an incomplete understanding of how different foods affect the body often lead to unhealthy food choices. Knowing what to eat, when to eat, and how to nourish the body with the right foods is essential for sustainable success. Understanding nutrition isn't just about cutting calories; it's about fueling your body in a way that supports health, energy, and weight loss.

Nowadays, the problem is not only a lack of knowledge, but also an overwhelming amount of misinformation. Social media is rife with self-proclaimed "coaches" offering health, nutrition, and exercise advice that lacks evidence or credibility. Conflicting information, such as Person A advocating for a no-carb diet, Person B promoting veganism, and Person C insisting on intermittent fasting, only leads to confusion and frustration. This highlights the importance of seeking accurate information from credible sources. As Coach Aizat frequently advises his clients, there is no one-size-fits-all "best" diet. Each person's optimal dietary approach is unique to their individual lifestyle and needs. Blindly following someone else's diet simply because it worked for them can lead to a frustrating cycle of yo-yo dieting.

5. **A Sedentary Lifestyle**

Obesity often develops as a result of a sedentary lifestyle, where physical activity is limited or nonexistent. Many people struggle to find ways to incorporate movement into their daily routines, whether it's because of time constraints or a lack of motivation. Exercise is essential for weight loss, but it must be something you enjoy. If exercise feels like a chore, it's much harder to stick with it.

Finding physical activities that you enjoy can make all the difference. Whether it's walking, dancing, swimming, or hiking, moving your body regularly is crucial to maintaining weight loss and improving overall health.

6. **Stress, Sleep, and Hormonal Imbalances**

Chronic stress, poor sleep, and hormonal imbalances all play significant roles in weight gain and weight loss struggles. Stress triggers emotional eating and cravings for unhealthy foods. Poor sleep affects the hormones that regulate hunger, making it harder to resist overeating.

Many people fail to recognize how much these factors impact their ability to lose weight. Addressing stress through relaxation techniques, ensuring adequate sleep, and managing hormones through diet and exercise are all key components of a holistic weight loss plan.

7. **Lack of Support**

Another reason why so many people fail to keep the weight off is the lack of support from friends, family, or a community. Going through the weight loss journey alone can be incredibly isolating. People who have a support system, whether it's a weight loss group, a friend, or a family member, are more likely to stay motivated and focused on their goals.

One powerful way to build support is by working with a coach. A coach provides personalized guidance, accountability, and expertise that can help navigate the challenges of weight loss. With a coach, you can set realistic goals, track your progress, and receive constant encouragement, which makes the journey more manageable. A coach also helps you stay committed, adjust your approach when necessary, and ensures you don't give up when faced with obstacles.

What Makes Sustained Success So Difficult?

The truth is, sustained weight loss success is difficult for a variety of reasons. Obesity is often deeply ingrained in our habits, environment, and even our psychology. Overcoming the hurdles of unhealthy eating habits, sedentary lifestyles, stress, and emotional eating requires more than just willpower. It requires a complete shift in mindset, a commitment to consistent action, and the willingness to address the deeper, often unspoken issues that contribute to weight gain.

Overcoming obesity is not just about losing weight—it's about transforming your entire approach to health and well-being. It's about creating a life where healthy choices are not just a temporary fix, but a permanent way of living.

In the earlier discussion, we explored the reasons why losing weight can be difficult. Now, let's continue by addressing one of the most common obstacles faced by overweight and obese individuals during the weight loss process: sustainability.

1. **Mismatch Between Prehistoric Human Body and Technological Advances in Society**

   As human beings evolved from hunters to organized societies, our metabolic system has remained largely unchanged, despite the tremendous technological advances in recent centuries. Diagram 3 on page 48, "Human Body Evolution vs. Technological Advances," illustrates the "mismatch gap" between the biological evolution of the human body and the rapid technological progress we've experienced. From the hunter-gatherer days to the rise of agricultural civilizations and later the industrial era, technological advancements have dramatically transformed how we live and work.

Today, many physical tasks that once required human effort, such as walking and manual labor, are now done by machines like cars, buses, trains, planes, and even robotic equipment in factories and workplaces. This shift has drastically reduced physical activity, with many people spending their workdays sitting in front of computers, assisted by artificial intelligence. This reduction in physical activity, both at work and during leisure time, has led to a significant caloric excess for millions of people. The excess calories are stored as body fat, contributing to obesity.

To overcome this mismatch, it is crucial for individuals to become aware of the impact of our modern lifestyles on our health. We must actively manage our calorie intake from food and drinks, balance it with our base metabolic rate (BMR), and increase our physical activity to ensure a caloric deficit that promotes fat burning and weight loss. This step is essential because our prehistoric ancestors' bodies were programmed to store excess calories as fat, a survival mechanism during times of starvation or famine. Unfortunately, this biological programming, once essential for survival, now works against us in an era of abundance and low physical activity.

As society advances technologically, our physical activity continues to decrease, and this trend will likely intensify with the development of even more advanced technologies. Therefore, it is vital to take intentional action to counteract the effects of this evolution mismatch.

Diagram 3: HUMAN BODY EVOLUTION VS TECHNOLOGICAL ADVANCES

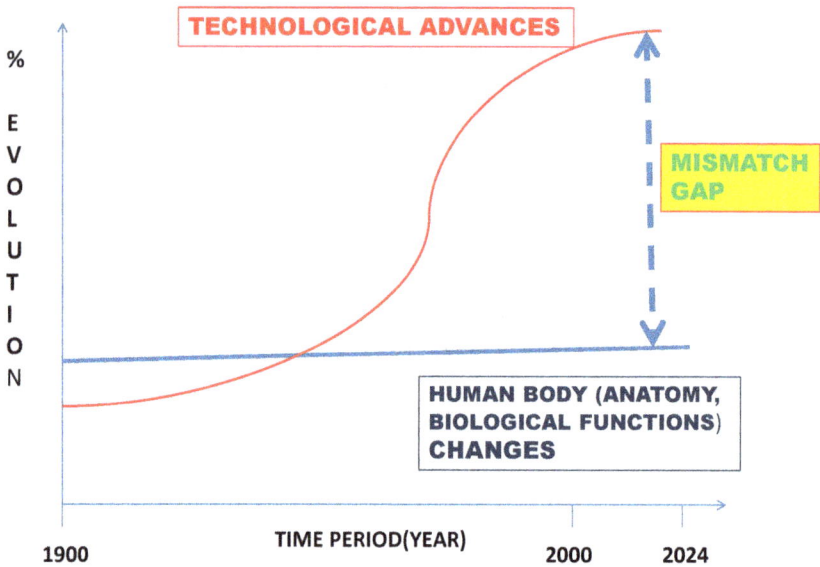

To make matters worse, the availability of cheap, processed junk food—typically high in calories—has drastically increased in comparison to early civilizations, where food was scarce and had to be hunted. Despite this shift in food availability, the human body still operates according to its prehistoric programming: it stores excess calories as body fat, a survival mechanism that helped our ancestors endure times of starvation and famine in challenging environments.

This creates a "double whammy" effect for modern humans: a tendency to overeat combined with a significant reduction in physical activity. Over time, this imbalance leads to an increase in body fat, contributing to obesity and overweight conditions.

2. **The Human Body as an Obstacle to Weight Loss and Maintenance**

As discussed in the previous section, the human body, shaped by prehistoric evolution, is programmed to store as much fat as possible for survival. This stored body fat serves as a reserve of energy in times of starvation or famine, a necessity during the early stages of human evolution millions of years ago.

Recent research supports the idea that our bodies biologically respond by gaining weight when they sense a significant loss of body fat. Two notable articles shed light on this phenomenon:

1. "Weighing the Facts: The Tough Truth About Weight Loss" by Marschall S. Runge, M.D., Ph.D., from Michigan Medicine, published on April 12, 2017.

2. "Unlocking the Secrets of Weight Regain: DNA Changes in Fat Cells May Explain Rebound Weight Gain" by Liveforever. club, quoting research led by Laura Catharina Hinte at the Swiss Federal Institute of Technology (ETH Zurich), published on November 18, 2024.

Dr. Runge's article highlights how biological changes, such as alterations in metabolism and hormonal signals, can work against weight loss efforts. When we lose weight, the body slows down our metabolism and releases hormones that trigger constant hunger, sending messages like "eat, eat, eat." Essentially, our body acts like an enemy, undermining our attempts to lose and maintain weight.

In the next chapters, we will explore how to build the mindset, habits, and systems necessary to conquer these challenges and achieve lasting success in the fight against obesity. Remember, the road to sustained weight loss is a journey—a journey that requires patience, perseverance, and the right strategies to succeed.

The Importance of a Holistic, Sustainable Approach

The key to overcoming these challenges is embracing a holistic approach to weight loss. This means considering not just what you eat or how much you exercise, but also how you manage stress, how you think about your body, and how you prioritize your health within the context of your busy life.

This book is rooted in the belief that sustainable weight loss is about more than just diet and exercise. It's about creating a lifestyle that promotes long-term health, resilience, and balance. It's about understanding that weight loss is a journey, not a quick fix. By addressing the physical, emotional, and mental barriers to weight loss, you can create lasting change.

The 6-Step System that we share in this book is designed to help you integrate these principles into your daily life, step by step, until they become second nature. It's about learning how to align your mind and body, manage stress, make time for health, and cultivate a positive mindset that empowers you to keep moving forward—no matter what challenges arise.

Ultimately, this book isn't just about losing weight; it's about transforming your life in a way that supports your health and well-being for years to come. It's a sustainable, holistic system that allows you to conquer obesity and build the foundation for a healthy, empowered life.

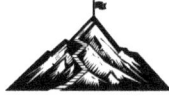

CHAPTER 1:

Cultivating a Positive Mindset for Weight Loss Success

The journey toward sustainable weight loss is far more than just a physical challenge; it's a mental and emotional one as well. To truly succeed, you must first cultivate a mindset that supports your goals. The power of belief is a fundamental key to achieving lasting change, and without it, even the most disciplined efforts can falter. In this chapter, we'll explore the power of belief, how to build a resilient, positive attitude, and techniques for maintaining motivation and sustaining momentum.

The Power of Belief in Achieving Weight Loss

Belief is one of the most powerful forces in shaping our reality. It dictates how we perceive challenges, how we approach setbacks, and ultimately how we achieve our goals. When it comes to weight loss, the belief that change is possible is critical. If you don't believe that you can lose weight and maintain a healthy lifestyle, your chances of success are significantly reduced.

"If you are faced with a mountain, you have several options. You can climb it and cross to the other side.

You can go around it. You can dig under it. You can fly over it. You can blow it up. You can ignore it and pretend it's not there. You can turn around and go back the way you came. Or you can stay on the mountain and make it your home."

— **Vera Nazarian**

The first step in cultivating a positive mindset for weight loss is recognizing that you are capable of change. It's important to understand that weight loss isn't just about changing your eating habits or your exercise routine—it's about transforming your mindset and embracing the process. Belief in your ability to succeed will keep you focused and resilient, even in the face of challenges.

Research has shown that people who believe they can lose weight are more likely to engage in the behaviors necessary for success. They're more likely to stick with their diet, prioritize exercise, and maintain the habits that lead to long-term results. On the other hand, a lack of belief often leads to self-sabotage, inconsistent efforts, and giving up after experiencing setbacks.

By developing a belief in your own abilities, you give yourself the foundation needed for lasting weight loss success. This belief empowers you to take action, stay committed, and handle challenges along the way.

Building a Resilient, Positive Attitude Toward Change

Resilience is the ability to bounce back after setbacks and keep moving forward despite obstacles. Building resilience is crucial for weight loss success because the path to achieving your goals will not always be smooth. There will be setbacks, temptations, and moments of doubt. How you handle these challenges can make or break your journey.

A resilient mindset involves reframing your thinking, especially when faced with obstacles. Instead of seeing a setback as a failure, view it as an opportunity to learn and grow. Did you slip up with your diet? It's okay. Instead of dwelling on guilt or disappointment, ask yourself what you can do differently next time. This shift in perspective allows you to keep moving forward without getting discouraged.

A positive attitude toward change is equally important. Often, we view change with apprehension or resistance, but adopting an attitude of openness and curiosity can make the process feel less daunting. Change doesn't have to be a battle—it can be an exciting journey. When you embrace the idea that each small step is progress, rather than focusing on the end result, the process becomes much more manageable.

Start by setting small, achievable goals and celebrating your victories along the way. Each time you hit a milestone—whether it's losing a few pounds, resisting a temptation, or sticking to your exercise routine—you reinforce your belief in your ability to succeed. Over time, these small successes build momentum and help you develop a resilient, positive attitude toward change.

Motivation Techniques and Sustaining Momentum

Motivation is the fuel that propels us toward our goals. However, it's important to recognize that motivation is not a constant force—it ebbs and flows. Some days, you may feel highly motivated and eager to make progress, while other days, the drive may feel completely absent. The key to long-term success, especially in a weight loss journey, is learning how to sustain that motivation, particularly on the tougher days when it seems more difficult to stay committed.

Maintaining momentum is about building practices and mindsets that help you push forward, even when you don't feel like it. By using the techniques outlined below, you can create a strong foundation that will keep you motivated through the inevitable ups and downs.

Visualize Your Success

Visualization is a powerful tool that successful individuals use to achieve their goals, and it can be especially effective in weight loss. Each day, take a few moments to vividly imagine yourself having already reached your weight loss goal. Picture yourself at your ideal weight or level of fitness, feeling energized, confident, and accomplished.

Think about the specific changes in your life that would occur once you achieve your goal: Perhaps you'll feel more comfortable in your clothes, be able to keep up with your children or grandchildren, or simply feel proud of yourself for accomplishing something significant. This mental image serves as a constant reminder of why you embarked on this journey in the first place, fueling your motivation to keep going, even when the going gets tough.

Visualization is not just about imagining your success, but also about how success will feel. How will you feel physically, emotionally, and mentally when you reach your weight loss goal? By frequently visualizing these positive outcomes, you reinforce your belief in what's possible and stay connected to the end result. This mental exercise can provide you with the energy and enthusiasm needed to face daily challenges.

Create a "Why" Statement

Coach Aizat's experience with numerous weight loss and fitness programs has revealed a key predictor of success: the strength of an individual's "big why." Those with a deeply personal and meaningful reason for weight loss, such as wanting to conceive, care for their physically-challenged loved ones, or see the wonders of the world, are more likely to succeed. Conversely, those with less compelling motivations, like an upcoming wedding or external pressure, often struggle.

Your "why" is the emotional and personal reason behind your desire to lose weight. It goes beyond wanting to fit into a smaller pair of jeans or look good on a beach—it's about understanding what motivates you at a deeper level. Your "why" is often linked to your core values, desires, and vision for your life.

Perhaps your "why" is about improving your health to avoid medical conditions, having the energy to enjoy family outings, or becoming more active so you can participate in physical activities you love. It might even be driven by a desire to feel more confident and comfortable in your own skin.

Take some time to write down your "why" statement. Be specific about what you're striving for and why it matters. For example, you might say, "I want to lose weight so I can be active with my kids without feeling winded, and so I can feel confident in my body again." Keep this statement visible—on your phone, on your fridge, or somewhere you'll see it regularly. When motivation wanes, revisiting your "why" can reignite your passion and keep you focused on what truly matters to you.

Break It Down into Small Steps

While your ultimate goal may be weight loss, focusing solely on that end result can feel overwhelming, especially when progress feels slow. Instead of fixating on a number on the scale or a distant date, break your goal into small, manageable steps.

Think of these small steps as the building blocks that will eventually get you to your larger goal. For example, aim to lose 1-2 pounds a week, rather than focusing on a larger, more daunting number. Celebrate each small victory along the way—whether it's drinking more water, walking an extra 10 minutes, or choosing a healthy meal option. Each small success is a step toward the bigger picture and serves as a reminder that you are making progress.

By focusing on daily or weekly goals, the process feels much more manageable. As you continue to check off these smaller goals, you'll build momentum, making it easier to stay motivated. These victories provide an immediate sense of accomplishment, helping you stay motivated even if the larger goal still feels far off.

Build Healthy Habits

Motivation can often feel fleeting. Some days, you'll wake up feeling inspired and ready to take on the world, but other days, it can be hard to muster the energy to work out or eat healthy. This is where habits come into play.

Habits are actions that become automatic over time, requiring less willpower and effort to maintain. The more you turn healthy behaviors into habits, the less you'll need to rely on motivation. This is a game-changer for long-term success.

Start by incorporating small, healthy habits into your daily routine. This could include things like meal prepping, scheduling workouts, or drinking water throughout the day. Once these actions become habits, they'll feel like second nature, and you won't have to force yourself to follow through. Over time, these small habits add up to big results, and you'll find yourself naturally moving closer to your weight loss goal, even when motivation is low.

Find Support and Accountability

Having support along your weight loss journey is crucial. It can be incredibly motivating to share your goals and progress with others who understand your challenges and celebrate your victories. Whether it's a friend, a family member, a workout buddy, or an online community, having someone to support you can make all the difference.

Support provides you with a network of encouragement and understanding, and it also creates a sense of accountability. When you know someone is expecting you to check in, work out, or stay on track with your meals, it's easier to stay committed. Accountability helps prevent you from skipping workouts or making unhealthy choices when nobody is watching.

Consider joining a group or finding a workout partner who shares similar goals. You can also hire a coach or health professional who can provide structured guidance and keep you on track. Share your progress regularly, celebrate milestones, and lean on each other when motivation is lacking.

Track Your Progress

Tracking your progress is a vital tool for staying motivated. It's easy to forget how far you've come when you're focused on what's left to achieve. Keeping a journal or using a weight loss app allows you to track your meals, workouts, and how you're feeling emotionally and physically throughout the process.

Tracking your progress not only helps you stay mindful of your actions, but it also provides you with a sense of accomplishment. You can see exactly how far you've come, even if the scale isn't moving as quickly as you'd like. This is especially important on days when you feel discouraged—your progress may not always show up on the scale, but tracking your habits can reveal how much you've improved overall.

It's also a great way to stay accountable. When you see your daily choices and behaviors in writing, you're more likely to stay consistent and make improvements where needed.

Be Kind to Yourself

Finally, it's essential to practice self-compassion. No one is perfect, and motivation can fluctuate. Some days, you may miss a workout, indulge in a treat, or skip a healthy meal. Instead of criticizing yourself or giving up entirely, practice kindness and patience.

Weight loss is a long-term journey, and setbacks are part of the process. Rather than focusing on guilt or shame, view these moments as opportunities to learn and adjust. Being kind to yourself helps you stay mentally and emotionally resilient, which is key to sustaining motivation over time.

Remember, the journey toward weight loss is not about being perfect—it's about progress. Embrace the ups and downs with a positive mindset and a commitment to keep moving forward, no matter how small the steps may seem.

Conclusion

A positive mindset is not just a "nice to have" when it comes to weight loss—it is one of the most powerful tools that will propel you toward success. The belief that you can achieve your goals is foundational to making progress. When you cultivate this mindset, you create an inner strength that allows you to face challenges with resilience and perseverance. It is this attitude that will help you stay motivated, even when obstacles arise or when the journey feels harder than expected.

Remember, weight loss is not just about the physical actions you take—what you believe and how you approach the process is just as important. The mental and emotional aspects of weight loss are often overlooked, but they are just as crucial to your success. A positive mindset shapes how you view challenges, how you cope with setbacks, and how you celebrate victories—both big and small.

When you adopt a positive mindset, you're not only setting yourself up for weight loss success, but also for a more fulfilling and empowered life. The confidence, resilience, and self-compassion you develop throughout this journey will extend beyond weight loss and positively impact other areas of your life. You'll find that the skills you build in the process—such as perseverance, discipline, and self-love—are the same ones that can help you succeed in all of your goals, whether they're personal, professional, or relational.

In the end, achieving your weight loss goals is about more than just changing your body—it's about transforming your mindset, your habits, and your life. With a positive mindset as your foundation, you will not only shed pounds, but also gain confidence, self-belief, and a sense of empowerment that lasts long after you've reached your target weight.

As you embrace this mindset, it's essential to recognize that stress can be one of the biggest obstacles in maintaining this positive outlook and staying on course. Stress can hinder your progress by triggering emotional eating, lowering motivation, and impacting your physical health. That's why in the next chapter, we will dive into *Managing Stress for Sustainable Weight Loss*. You'll learn effective strategies to manage stress, reduce its impact on your body, and ensure that it doesn't derail your weight loss journey. Let's explore how to transform stress into a tool for resilience, rather than a barrier.

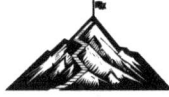

Chapter 2:

Managing Stress for Sustainable Weight Loss

"When preparing to climb a mountain – pack a light heart."

—Dan May

In our pursuit of a healthier life, stress often feels like an unrelenting force that challenges our well-being. It takes many forms—work pressures, relationship struggles, financial concerns—and can affect us emotionally, mentally, and physically. The weight of these stressors can leave us overwhelmed and drained, making it hard to find balance.

But have you ever considered how stress might not only impact your emotions but also your physical health and weight management? Chronic stress can disrupt your body's natural processes, including hormones, sleep patterns, and metabolism, ultimately influencing your ability to lose or maintain weight. Stress increases cortisol, a hormone linked to fat storage, particularly around the abdomen, and can trigger emotional eating, cravings for unhealthy foods, and a sedentary lifestyle—all of which undermine your weight loss goals.

In this chapter, we will explore the intricate relationship between stress and weight loss. We'll examine how the physiological and psychological effects of stress can sabotage even the most well-intentioned efforts to achieve a healthy weight. However, we won't just focus on the challenges—we will also provide practical strategies to manage stress, build resilience, and maintain balance in your life.

By cultivating a mindful approach to stress and incorporating healthy coping mechanisms, you'll be empowered to manage stress in ways that support both your mental and physical health. With these tools, you can create a sustainable path toward weight loss that prioritizes overall well-being, not just the number on the scale. Together, we'll unlock the keys to a more balanced and healthier life—no longer held hostage by stress, but mastering it to thrive.

The Stress-Weight Connection

To manage stress effectively, it's essential to understand its profound connection to weight management. Chronic stress doesn't just affect how we feel emotionally—it directly impacts our physical health and metabolism. Research shows that stress disrupts our hormonal balance, leading to a cascade of negative effects on both our health and weight.

Cortisol, the "stress hormone," is a primary factor in this process. During stressful moments, the body releases cortisol as part of the fight-or-flight response. In the short term, this is protective, but chronic stress causes sustained high cortisol levels, which can disrupt metabolism and promote fat storage, particularly around the abdomen. Elevated cortisol levels are strongly linked to an increased risk of heart disease, diabetes, and other metabolic disorders.

Stress also triggers cravings for high-calorie comfort foods, rich in sugar, fat, and salt. These cravings are linked to how stress impacts our brain's reward system. When we consume these foods, our brains release dopamine, a "feel-good" neurotransmitter, providing temporary relief from stress. However, this relief often leads to overeating, creating a cycle of emotional eating that undermines weight management.

Furthermore, stress depletes our mental energy, making it harder to stick to healthy habits. It clouds decision-making abilities and weakens our motivation, making it more difficult to prioritize nutritious meals or exercise. The fatigue from constant stress can leave us feeling drained, turning healthy choices into burdens.

Over time, emotional eating can become a habitual coping mechanism. Instead of addressing the root causes of stress, we may turn to food for comfort, numbing emotional discomfort without resolving the underlying issues. This behavior not only sabotages weight loss but also diminishes overall well-being.

The key to overcoming the stress-weight connection is awareness. By recognizing how stress affects both our body and behavior, we can make mindful choices that support our health and weight management. In the next section, we'll explore practical techniques for managing stress, helping you break free from the cycle of emotional eating and regain control of both your stress and weight.

Building Resilience: Practical Techniques for Overcoming Stress

To overcome the negative impact of stress on our weight management journey, it is crucial to build resilience. Resilience acts as a shield, helping us navigate life's challenges while maintaining our focus on healthier choices. It empowers us to recover from setbacks and continue making positive decisions, even when facing stress. Here are some practical techniques to cultivate resilience and maintain balance in your life:

1. **Mindful Meditation:** Mindful meditation is one of the most effective ways to manage stress. By dedicating time each day to focus on your breath, thoughts, and bodily sensations, you enhance your ability to remain calm and present. This practice promotes self-awareness, allowing you to better identify and address stress triggers before they escalate. Regular mindfulness practice can reduce anxiety, help you make thoughtful decisions, and enable you to respond to stress in a calm, controlled manner. Even just a few minutes of meditation daily can foster emotional stability and mental clarity.

2. **Exercise as Stress Relief:** Physical activity is not just beneficial for your body; it also serves as a powerful stress-reliever. Exercise triggers the release of endorphins, the body's natural mood boosters, which can alleviate anxiety and improve overall mood. It also promotes healthy blood circulation, which boosts energy levels and promotes well-being. Whether it's jogging, dancing, yoga, or another form of movement, find an activity you genuinely enjoy, and make it a regular part of your routine. Consistent exercise helps you build both physical strength and mental resilience, which is key to overcoming stress and maintaining a healthy weight.

3. **Prioritize Self-Care:** In the chaos of daily life, self-care often takes a backseat, but it is an essential aspect of building resilience. Make self-care a priority by ensuring you get adequate sleep, nourish your body with healthy food, and take time for activities that bring you joy. This may include reading, cooking, or spending time outdoors. Self-care is an investment in your physical, emotional, and mental health, and it ensures you have the energy and mindset needed to tackle life's challenges. Remember, prioritizing self-care is not indulgent; it is necessary for long-term well-being.

4. **Connect with Supportive Individuals:** Building a network of supportive friends, family members, or even joining a weight loss or wellness community can be instrumental in navigating challenging times. Surround yourself with people who motivate, inspire, and understand you. These individuals offer not only encouragement but also a safe space for expressing your feelings and releasing stress. By connecting with others who share similar goals or experiences, you can foster a sense of belonging and receive the emotional support necessary to stay on track.

5. **Explore Stress-Relieving Strategies:** Stress relief is not one-size-fits-all, so it's important to discover which methods work best for you. Engaging in hobbies, practicing deep breathing exercises, or seeking professional help, such as therapy or counseling, can provide relief. If you enjoy creative outlets, consider painting, writing, or crafting as a way to express and release built-up emotions. Explore different techniques until you find what brings you a sense of calm and balance. Remember, stress-relief strategies are essential not just for weight management but for overall mental health.

6. **Cognitive Restructuring:** Our thoughts significantly influence how we respond to stress. Cognitive restructuring is the practice of identifying negative or distorted thought patterns and replacing them with more positive and realistic perspectives. This can be especially helpful when managing stress and preventing it from negatively impacting your weight loss journey. Start by recognizing self-limiting thoughts and challenge them. For example, if you think "I can't handle this," reframe it with "I've overcome challenges before, and I can do it again." Positive affirmations and thought reframing can help you approach stress with a more resilient mindset.

7. **Time Management:** When responsibilities pile up and time feels limited, stress can intensify. Effective time management is key to reducing overwhelm and creating a sense of control. Start by prioritizing tasks based on importance and urgency, breaking them down into smaller, manageable steps. Delegate tasks where possible, and ensure you schedule breaks to recharge. Setting realistic goals and boundaries is essential in maintaining balance. Remember, it's okay to say no when necessary—it's a form of self-care that can help you avoid burnout and maintain focus on your priorities.

8. **Journaling:** Writing down your thoughts, feelings, and experiences can serve as a powerful tool for managing stress. Journaling provides a safe space for self-expression and emotional release, reducing the intensity of stress and promoting reflection. Consider keeping a gratitude journal where you write down three things you are thankful for every day. This simple practice helps shift your focus toward the positive, enhancing resilience and providing a sense of perspective during difficult times.

9. **Relaxation Techniques:** Incorporating relaxation techniques into your daily routine can significantly reduce stress and promote overall well-being. Techniques such as deep breathing exercises, progressive muscle relaxation, or guided imagery can help you unwind and recharge. Make it a habit to engage in these practices regularly, especially during times of heightened stress. Over time, relaxation techniques can lower cortisol levels, improve sleep quality, and help you feel more grounded and centered.

10. **Finding Joy and Laughter:** Stress often makes life feel heavy, but moments of joy and laughter can be powerful antidotes. Engaging in activities that bring you happiness and surrounding yourself with people who make you laugh can drastically reduce stress. Laughter releases endorphins, the body's natural feel-good chemicals, which help reduce stress hormones, lower blood pressure, and boost the immune system. Whether it's watching a funny movie, spending time with loved ones, or indulging in a favorite hobby, finding joy and laughter regularly can have a profound positive impact on both your physical and mental health.

By integrating these practical techniques into your life, you can build resilience against stress and create a sustainable foundation for maintaining both emotional balance and physical well-being. Resilience enables you to face challenges with confidence, make empowered choices, and continue progressing toward your weight management and wellness goals.

Conclusion

Managing stress is an essential aspect of achieving sustainable weight loss. Stress not only affects our mental and emotional health but also has a direct impact on our physical well-being, including our ability to manage weight. By understanding how stress influences our eating habits, hormones, and energy levels, we can take proactive steps to mitigate its effects and stay on track toward our goals.

As we wrap up this chapter, it's important to acknowledge that managing stress is not a one-time task; rather, it is a continuous process. Just like weight loss, mastering stress management requires patience, persistence, and practice. You may experience both progress and setbacks along the way, and that's okay. The key is to approach the process with self-compassion, understanding that each step you take is part of your overall growth.

As you continue to build resilience and develop healthier stress responses, remember that stress management is not a destination—it's a journey. By incorporating these techniques into your daily routine, you're investing in your long-term well-being. With each day of practice, you become better equipped to handle life's challenges without letting stress interfere with your health goals.

Stay committed to your well-being, and continue to embrace each phase of your journey. With the tools and resilience you've gained, you're well on your way to achieving a healthier, more balanced life. The path to sustainable weight loss may not always be straightforward, but with each step, you are building the strength and mindset necessary to thrive. You are capable of achieving the healthy, vibrant life you deserve.

As we move forward, another critical aspect of your weight loss journey comes into play—time management. Balancing the demands of daily life with the time and energy required for weight loss can be challenging, but with the right approach, it is entirely possible. In the next chapter, *Optimizing Time Management for Weight Loss*, we will explore strategies to make the most of your time, helping you stay consistent with healthy habits and prioritize your well-being without feeling overwhelmed. Let's dive into how you can manage your time effectively and make your weight loss journey a more manageable and sustainable part of your daily life.

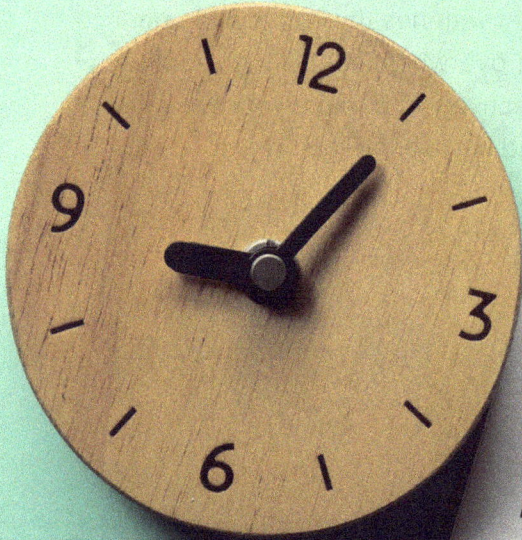

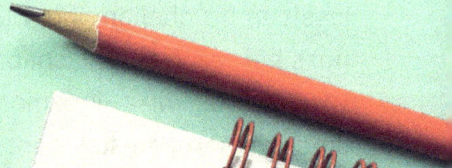

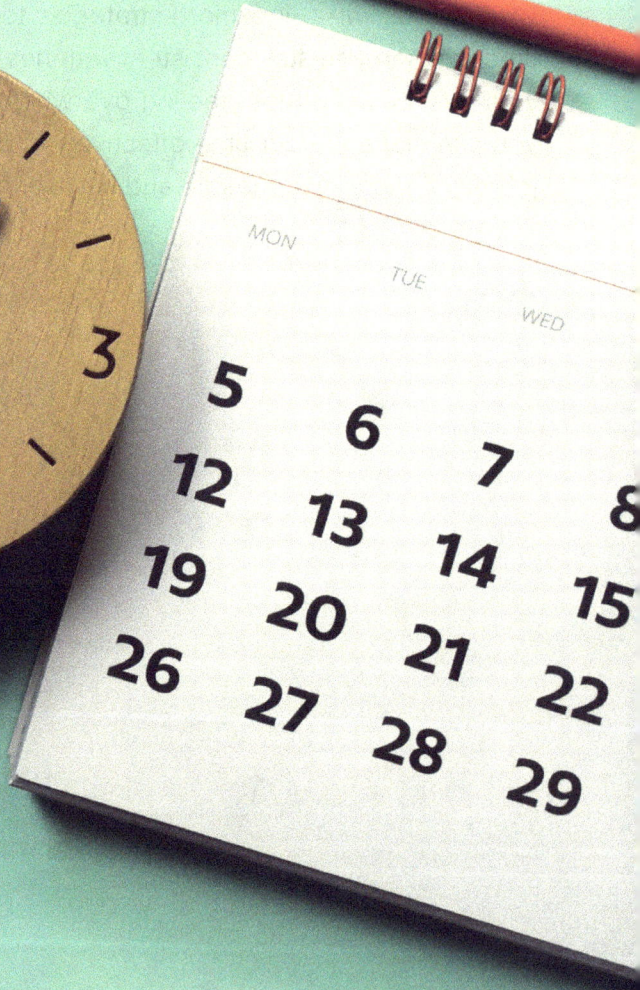

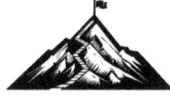

CHAPTER 3:

Optimizing Time Management for Weight Loss

"Be prepared to climb one kilometer more. The way up to the top of the mountain is always longer than you think. Don't fool yourself, the moment will arrive when what seemed so near is still very far."

—Paulo Coelho

For many, time appears to be the greatest barrier to weight loss. Work deadlines, family responsibilities, and social obligations often take precedence, leaving little room for meal preparation, exercise, or self-care. However, the truth is that no one "finds" time for wellness—they create it.

"I don't have the time. My work is exhausting, and by the time I get home, I just want to rest. I have kids to take care of."

Does this sound familiar? I've been there too. But let me ask you:

- Do you watch TV?

- Do you scroll through TikTok, Facebook, or Instagram?

If you answered yes, you're likely spending at least two hours a day on these activities. That adds up to 60 hours a month and 730 hours a year.

Now, let's revisit the question. Do you really not have the time?

The truth is, you do. The real issue is how you prioritize your time. We often prioritize what offers short-term comfort over what truly benefits our health and long-term well-being.

But here's the good news: This pattern can be changed. Small shifts in how you manage your time can lead to life-changing results. The choice is yours. Will you continue chasing temporary relief, or will you invest in your long-term health and strength?

In today's fast-paced world, time has become one of our most precious resources. When it comes to reaching weight loss goals and achieving optimal well-being, effective time management is crucial. By recognizing the value of time in our weight loss journey, we can make the most of every moment and put our health first.

To shift this narrative, health-related activities must no longer be viewed as optional but rather as non-negotiable investments in oneself. A healthier you is more productive, more energetic, and better equipped to handle life's demands.

Time is a finite resource, and how you choose to utilize it can make all the difference in achieving weight loss goals. Unfortunately, many people inadvertently waste valuable time on activities that do not contribute to their well-being and distract them from the ultimate goal of lasting weight loss.

Identifying Time Traps

Before optimizing your time management for weight loss, it's crucial to identify the time traps that often derail progress. Time traps are activities or habits that consume your time without offering meaningful benefits. These unproductive patterns and distractions can create significant obstacles to achieving your weight loss and wellness goals. By recognizing and addressing these time traps, you can channel your energy toward healthier, more productive actions. Common culprits include procrastination, unproductive multitasking, and mindless activities.

Procrastination

Procrastination is one of the most pervasive time traps, often fueled by a lack of motivation, fear of failure, or feelings of being overwhelmed. It's the act of postponing important activities, such as preparing nutritious meals or exercising, under the false belief that you'll "get to it later." Unfortunately, "later" often turns into "never," leaving you with a growing sense of guilt and a lack of progress.

Why It Impacts Weight Loss:

- **Leads to missed opportunities for essential health habits:** Skipping workouts or opting for unhealthy takeout due to procrastination directly sabotages your weight loss efforts. **Increases stress:** As tasks pile up, stress levels rise, which can trigger emotional eating. The accumulation of undone tasks often leads to unhealthy comfort food choices, contributing to weight gain.

- **Undermines confidence:** Repeatedly putting off healthy behaviors erodes your self-efficacy, making it harder to believe in and commit to future weight loss goals.

- **Disrupted routine and inconsistent progress:** Procrastination makes it difficult to establish a consistent routine, leading to sporadic efforts that hinder steady progress.

- **Reduced motivation and increased frustration:** The cycle of procrastination and guilt can fuel feelings of frustration and demotivation, making it even harder to get back on track.

How to Overcome Procrastination:

1. **Break Tasks into Bite-Sized Pieces:** Tackling a smaller portion of a task makes it feel less daunting. For example, instead of planning a week's worth of meals, start by prepping just one meal.

2. **Set a Timer:** Use a timer to commit to just 10-15 minutes of focused effort. Often, starting is the hardest part, and once you begin, you'll find it easier to keep going.

3. **Focus on the Rewards:** Remind yourself how you'll feel after completing the task—whether it's the satisfaction of a healthy meal or the endorphins from a workout.

4. **Prioritize and Schedule:** Identify the most important tasks and schedule them into your day. This helps avoid decision fatigue and ensures that essential activities don't get pushed aside.

5. **Eliminate Distractions:** Create a focused environment by minimizing distractions like social media, email, or television.

This allows you to fully engage in the task at hand and complete it more efficiently.

6. **Find an Accountability Partner:** Share your goals with a friend or family member who can check in on your progress and provide support. Knowing that someone is aware of your commitments can help you stay motivated and accountable.

7. **Forgive Yourself and Move On:** If you do procrastinate (we are humans after all), don't dwell on it. Acknowledge the lapse, forgive yourself, and recommit to your goals. Remember that progress, not perfection, is the key.

Unproductive Multitasking

While multitasking might seem like a way to maximize time, it often has the opposite effect. Dividing your attention between multiple tasks reduces your focus and efficiency, leaving you with subpar results. For instance, trying to prep meals while responding to emails might lead to mistakes, wasted ingredients, or even accidents in the kitchen.

Why It Hurts Progress:

- Reduces the quality of your efforts, such as half-hearted workouts or poorly prepared meals.

- Leads to more time spent correcting mistakes or redoing tasks.

- Creates mental fatigue, making it harder to stay motivated throughout the day.

- Increases stress and anxiety due to the feeling of constantly juggling tasks.

- Impairs memory and cognitive function, making it harder to retain information and learn new skills.

- Decreases productivity by hindering your ability to fully engage in any one task.

- Can lead to unhealthy food choices if you're distracted during meal times and not paying attention to what you're eating.

Strategies to Minimize Multitasking:

1. **Prioritize Tasks:** Identify the most critical health-related activities and tackle them one at a time.

2. **Use Focus Blocks:** Dedicate specific periods to single tasks, like a 30-minute workout or a 20-minute meal prep session.

3. **Eliminate Distractions:** Turn off notifications, mute your phone, or use apps that block access to distracting websites during focused activities.

4. **Create a Dedicated Workspace:** If possible, designate a specific area for tasks like meal prep or exercise. This helps minimize distractions and enhances focus.

5. **Set Realistic Goals:** Avoid overloading yourself with too many tasks at once. Start with manageable goals and gradually increase them as you build focus and discipline.

6. **Practice Mindfulness:** Cultivate present-moment awareness to stay focused on the task at hand and avoid the urge to switch between activities.

7. **Take Breaks:** Schedule short breaks between focus blocks to refresh your mind and avoid burnout.

Mindless Activities

Mindless activities are perhaps the most insidious time traps, often going unnoticed until hours have slipped away. Scrolling through social media, binge-watching TV shows, or playing mobile games may feel relaxing in the moment, but these activities rarely contribute to your overall well-being. In fact, excessive screen time can leave you feeling more fatigued, disconnected, and unmotivated.

How It Sabotages Wellness:

- Steals time that could be spent on exercise, meal preparation, or relaxation.

- Reinforces sedentary behavior, which is counterproductive to weight loss.

- Contributes to decision fatigue, leaving you less capable of making healthy choices later in the day.

- Can lead to mindless eating and overconsumption of unhealthy snacks.

- Disrupts sleep patterns if done close to bedtime, affecting energy levels and cravings.

- Negatively impacts mental health by promoting comparison and feelings of inadequacy.

Ways to Reduce Mindless Activities:

1. **Set Screen Time Limits:** Use apps or built-in phone features to cap your time on social media or streaming platforms.

2. **Replace with Active Breaks:** Instead of scrolling during downtime, take a 5- to 10-minute walk or stretch to boost energy and burn calories.

3. **Be Intentional with Leisure Time:** Plan your entertainment in advance—choose a single show or allocate a specific amount of time to social media.

4. **Create Tech-Free Zones:** Designate specific areas or times of day where technology is off-limits, such as during meals or before bed.

5. **Find Alternative Hobbies:** Explore new hobbies that engage your mind and body, such as reading, cooking, gardening, or learning a new skill.

6. **Digital Detox:** Occasionally disconnect completely from technology for a set period to recharge and reconnect with yourself and your surroundings.

Reclaiming Your Time

By addressing procrastination, unproductive multitasking, and mindless activities, you can reclaim hours in your day and redirect them toward meaningful, health-promoting actions. These small adjustments to how you manage your time can have a profound impact on your ability to stay consistent, achieve weight loss goals, and maintain a balanced lifestyle. Remember, every moment is an opportunity—make it count.

Creating a Personalized Health Schedule

Now that we recognize the value of time and understand the time traps we may encounter, it's time to take control and create a personalized health schedule. By carefully managing our time, we can ensure that we allocate appropriate slots for exercise, meal preparation, and self-care.

A well-structured schedule is key to integrating health-related activities seamlessly into your daily routine, making them feel like second nature rather than a chore. By following these steps, you can create a personalized schedule that aligns with your weight loss goals and lifestyle:

1. **Assess Your Current Routine**

Start with a time audit to gain a clear understanding of how you currently spend your day. Use tools like a planner or time-tracking app to log your activities for a few days. Identify time gaps or periods where you might be engaging in unproductive activities, such as excessive screen time, that could instead be used for wellness tasks.

2. **Set Clear Priorities**

Determine which health-related activities—like exercise, meal preparation, or relaxation—are most important for achieving your goals. Prioritize these activities based on their impact. For example, if regular workouts are essential to your plan, they should take precedence in your schedule.

3. **Block Specific Time Slots**

Time blocking is an effective strategy for ensuring health-related activities are part of your day. Allocate dedicated time for tasks such as meal prep, exercise, or meditation. Treat these blocks as unmovable appointments with yourself. For example:

- **Morning:** Schedule a quick workout or mindfulness session before starting your workday.

- **Evening:** Reserve time for meal prep or a calming routine to wind down.

4. **Build in Flexibility**

Life is unpredictable, and rigid schedules can feel overwhelming. Incorporate buffer times or alternative options into your plan. For instance, if a meeting runs late, a 10-minute evening walk could replace a full workout. This flexibility ensures that setbacks don't derail your progress.

5. **Use Tools to Stay on Track**

Leverage digital tools like calendars, alarms, or habit-tracking apps to remind you of your scheduled activities. Visualizing your commitments can help you stay accountable and focused.

By carefully structuring your day with these strategies, health-related activities can become ingrained habits, helping you maintain consistent progress toward your weight loss and wellness goals.

Sample Health Schedule

Here's an example of how a health-focused day might look:

- **Morning (7:00–7:30 AM):** A quick workout, stretching, or yoga to energize your day.

- **Lunch Break (12:00–12:15 PM):** A short walk around the block to refresh and boost circulation.

- **Evening (6:00–6:30 PM):** Prepare a nutritious dinner or engage in light meal prep for the following day.

Finding Micro-Moments for Wellness

Micro-moments, those tiny intervals throughout the day, may seem insignificant, but they can have a tremendous impact on your weight loss journey. These moments are the windows of opportunity to incorporate healthy habits into your daily routine. Whether it's taking the stairs instead of the elevator, doing squats while waiting for your coffee, or practicing deep breathing during a stressful moment, seizing these micro-moments for wellness can be transformative.

The key to optimizing your time management is to be mindful and aware of these opportunities. By consciously seeking out these micro-moments, you can squeeze in extra physical activity, mindfulness, or healthy choices that contribute to your weight loss goals.

Every moment counts on your journey to lasting weight loss. By understanding the value of time, identifying your time traps, creating a personalized health schedule, and finding micro-moments for wellness, you can optimize your time management for weight loss and enhance your overall well-being.

Maximizing Time Efficiency for Weight Loss

Now that we have laid the foundation of understanding the value of time management in our weight loss journey, and have recognized the time traps we often fall into, it's time to delve deeper into techniques and strategies for optimizing our time efficiency.

Identifying and eliminating time traps is a crucial step, but it's equally important to make the most of the time we have available. With our busy lives, it can be challenging to find enough hours in the day for exercise, healthy meal preparation, and self-care. However, with intentional planning and prioritization, we can make it happen.

Batch Cooking and Meal Planning

One effective time management tool for weight loss is batch cooking and meal planning. Dedicate a specific time each week to plan and prepare your meals for the upcoming days. This not only saves time but also ensures that you have nutritious, pre-prepared meals readily available, eliminating the need for unhealthy last-minute choices.

Consider setting aside a few hours on the weekends to cook in bulk. Prepare a variety of lean proteins, whole grains, and vegetables that can be easily combined into different meals throughout the week. Divide them into portion-controlled containers for grab-and-go convenience. By doing this, you save time on meal preparation during busy weekdays while staying in control of your nutrition.

Learning to Say No

Another aspect of time management often overlooked is learning to say no. As individuals striving for weight loss and optimal well-being, it's essential to prioritize our health and set boundaries. This means saying no to activities, events, or commitments that do not align with our goals or compromise our time for self-care and exercise.

It can be challenging, but it's important to remember that saying no to certain things allows us to say yes to our health. This means politely declining invitations to social gatherings that revolve around unhealthy food and drink choices or restructuring our daily routines to make time for physical activity. By setting boundaries and prioritizing our well-being, we ensure that our time is used effectively, and our weight loss goals come to fruition.

Utilizing Technology to Optimize Time

While excessive screen time can be a time trap, technology can also be a valuable tool in optimizing our time management for weight loss. With numerous health and fitness apps available, we can track our progress, access workout routines, and receive motivation and support.

Consider exploring these apps and finding ones that align with your goals and preferences. Some apps offer guided workouts for different fitness levels, provide nutrition tracking, and even send reminders to ensure you stay on track. By incorporating technology into our weight loss journey, we can streamline our efforts and make the most of our time.

Leveraging Support Systems

We often underestimate the power of a support system when it comes to weight loss and time management. Surrounding ourselves with like-minded individuals who share similar goals can provide motivation, accountability, and valuable insights.

Find a workout buddy or join a weight loss support group either online or in person. These connections can help you stay committed and inspired, as well as offer tips on time-saving strategies that have worked for them. Sharing experiences and challenges with others who understand can make a significant difference in your weight loss journey.

Maintaining Balance and Flexibility

While optimizing time management for weight loss is crucial, it's also important to maintain a healthy balance and flexibility. Life can sometimes throw unexpected curveballs, and it's crucial to adapt and adjust our schedules accordingly.

Be kind to yourself and understand that there may be days when your time doesn't align perfectly with your weight loss goals. Embrace flexibility and focus on making the best choices possible in those moments. Remember, it's the long-term consistency that matters most for lasting weight loss and well-being.

Incorporating Mindfulness Practices

When managing our time, we often focus solely on the practical aspects of weight loss. However, incorporating mindfulness practices can significantly enhance our overall well-being, boost our motivation, and reduce stress levels.

Take a few moments each day to practice mindfulness and be present in the current moment. This can be as simple as practicing deep breathing exercises, meditating for a few minutes, or engaging in mindful eating. By incorporating mindfulness, we cultivate a sense of awareness and appreciation for the choices we make, leading to more intentional time management and improved weight loss outcomes.

Conclusion

Optimizing time management for weight loss is no easy feat, but with the right strategies and a commitment to prioritizing your health, it becomes entirely achievable. Every moment counts, and by implementing the techniques outlined in this chapter— leveraging micro-moments, planning meals efficiently, utilizing technology, setting boundaries, and embracing mindfulness— you can take control of your time and make measurable progress toward your weight loss and well-being goals.

Stay consistent, be kind to yourself, and celebrate the small victories that pave the way for lasting success. Remember, weight loss and optimal health are lifelong pursuits, not quick fixes. Cultivating a positive relationship with time and building habits that align with your goals will ensure that your journey is sustainable and fulfilling.

As you progress along this journey, it's important to remember that healthy living is not just about managing time effectively or focusing on one aspect of wellness—it's about embracing a holistic approach. In the next chapter, we'll delve into *The 8 Key Elements of Healthy Living*, which are crucial for achieving sustainable weight loss and overall well-being. These elements will give you a broader perspective on health and help you establish a solid foundation that supports not just weight loss, but a vibrant, balanced life. By focusing on these essential aspects of your health, you'll be empowered to take charge of your overall wellness in a way that supports lasting success. Let's explore how these key elements can transform your approach to healthy living.

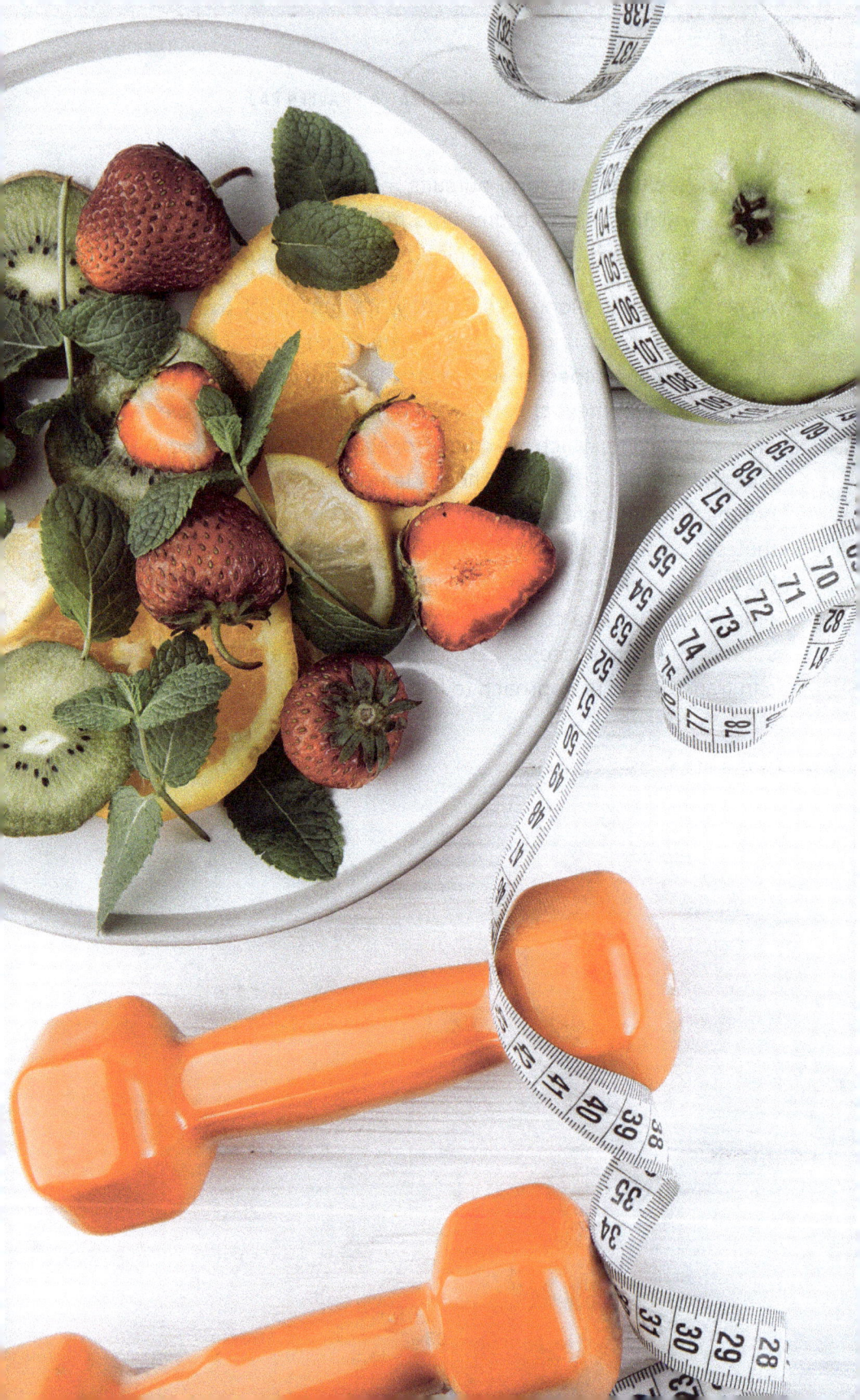

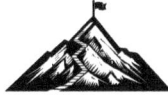

CHAPTER 4:

The 8 Essential Elements of Healthy Living

"Mountains know secrets we need to learn. That might take time, it might be hard, but if you just hold on long enough, you will find the strength to rise up."

—Tyler Knott

Achieving sustainable weight loss is not a simple, linear process. It requires a holistic approach that encompasses various aspects of your life. The 6-Step System requires understanding the interconnectivity of various elements that affect the weight loss process. Diagram 4 on page 88 illustrates the 8 Essential Elements of Healthy Living, providing a comprehensive framework to help you understand the key aspects of each element and how they contribute to achieving your weight loss goals while maintaining a balanced, healthy, and safe lifestyle. These elements are divided into two groups: the inner six elements, which focus on your physical and mental healthy living, and the outer two elements, which focus on personal safety culture. With sufficient understanding and knowledge of the 8 elements and, committing to them is essential as you embark on your weight loss journey, creating an environment conducive to a healthy, safe and successful life. By integrating them into your daily routine, you create a sustainable foundation for lasting results. Let's explore each element and how it contributes to your overall health, personal safety and weight loss success.

Diagram 4: The 8 Essential Elements of Healthy Living

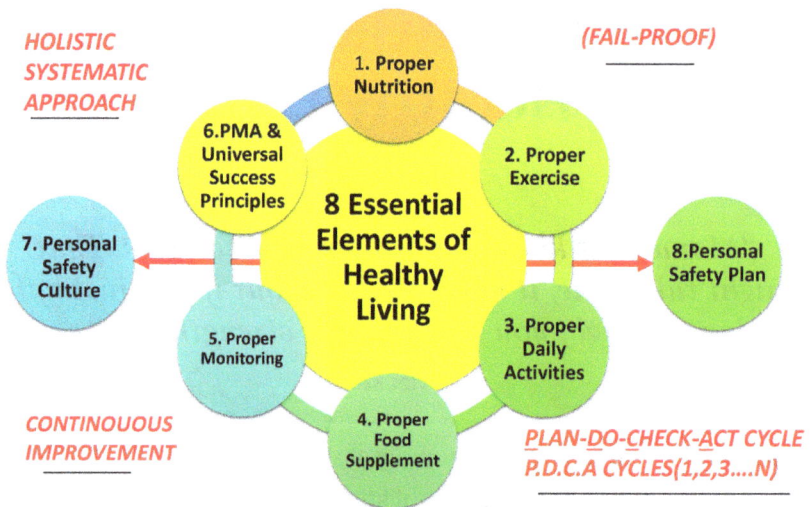

HOLISTIC SYSTEMATIC APPROACH

(FAIL-PROOF)

1. Proper Nutrition

6.PMA & Universal Success Principles

2. Proper Exercise

8 Essential Elements of Healthy Living

7. Personal Safety Culture

8.Personal Safety Plan

5. Proper Monitoring

3. Proper Daily Activities

CONTINOUOUS IMPROVEMENT

4. Proper Food Supplement

PLAN-DO-CHECK-ACT CYCLE P.D.C.A CYCLES(1,2,3....N)

Element 1: Proper Nutrition

Nutrition is the cornerstone of good health and weight management. It's not just about what you eat but how it fuels your body and supports your energy levels. Proper nutrition provides the essential nutrients your body needs to function optimally, and understanding the impact of your food choices can make a significant difference in your weight loss outcomes.

Principles of Proper Nutrition

- **Eat to live, not live to eat:** Focus on nourishing your body rather than indulging in food as a source of comfort or entertainment.

- **Moderation is key:** Strive for a balanced diet, avoiding extremes and ensuring you consume adequate nutrients without overeating.

- **Be mindful of your body's needs:** Your body has specific nutritional requirements, and it's important to understand what works best for your individual health and wellness goals.

Basic 101

Proper nutrition includes:

- **Macronutrients:** Proteins, fats, and carbohydrates provide your body with energy.

- **Micronutrients:** Vitamins and minerals are essential for cellular functions and overall health.

- **Water:** Hydration is crucial for every bodily function, including digestion and circulation.

- **Fiber:** This aids in digestion and prevents chronic diseases.

Knowing the principles of energy balance:

Macronutrients—protein, carbohydrates, and fats—provide your body with energy, measured in calories (kcal). Protein and carbs offer 4 kcal per gram, while fats provide 9 kcal per gram. This constitutes your energy intake or "calories in." Your energy output, or "calories out," is the energy your body uses daily, also known as Total Daily Energy Expenditure (TDEE).

Your TDEE comprises three primary factors:

- **~70% Basal Metabolic Rate (BMR)**: Calories burned at rest to sustain essential bodily functions. BMR is influenced by age, gender, muscle mass, and genetics.

- **~15% Non-Exercise Activity Thermogenesis (NEAT)**: Calories burned through daily activities like walking, fidgeting, or chores.

- **~5% Exercise Activity Thermogenesis (EAT)**: Calories burned during structured exercise or workouts.

- **~10% Thermic Effect of Feeding (TEF)**: Energy used to digest, absorb, and process food. Protein has a higher TEF (20-30%) than carbohydrates (5-10%) and fats (0-3%).

While factors like genetics, age, and gender are uncontrollable, you can influence your daily calorie burn by increasing muscle mass by doing resistance training and getting enough protein, doing cardiovascular exercise (jogging, cycling and swimming), increasing your daily steps, and even choosing extra protein also significantly helps with your weight loss journey.

Weight management revolves around energy balance: calories consumed versus calories used. Maintaining weight means calorie intake equals calorie expenditure. To lose weight, create a calorie deficit by consuming fewer calories than you burn. For instance, if you burn 2,000 calories daily, consuming 1,600 calories creates a deficit. Body fat stores excess energy; a calorie surplus leads to fat storage, while a deficit prompts the body to use stored fat for energy.

Understanding energy balance is fundamental for weight management. Calculate your TDEE using online calculators and employ strategies to manage calorie intake and output. Remember that individual needs and lifestyles vary, so find what works best for you to achieve a calorie deficit.

Actions

- Create a caloric deficit of around 250-500 calories per day for gradual weight loss. You might think a bigger calorie deficit is better, however it is unhealthy, especially done long-term.

- Reduce consumption of fried foods and sugary drinks, opting for healthier alternatives like whole fruits, vegetables, and lean proteins.

- Consider incorporating intermittent fasting to boost metabolism and enhance mental clarity.

- If needed, consult a nutritionist or dietitian for personalized advice on balancing your macronutrients.

- Increase your protein intake to promote satiety and preserve muscle mass.

- Focus on whole, unprocessed foods and limit refined carbohydrates.

- Practice portion control and mindful eating to avoid overeating.

- Stay hydrated by drinking plenty of water throughout the day.

- Limit alcohol consumption, as it can contribute empty calories and hinder weight loss.

- Get adequate sleep, as sleep deprivation can disrupt hormones that regulate hunger and metabolism.

Element 2: Proper Exercise

Exercise is an essential part of maintaining overall health. It not only helps with weight management but also supports mental well-being, energy levels, and cognitive function. Exercise can take many forms, it is essential to do ones that are based on your ability and fitness level. Besides that, the key to long-term exercise habits is to engage in activities that you enjoy and that fit your lifestyle.

Principles of Proper Exercise

- Exercise enhances strength, flexibility, and balance, leading to improved physical function and reduced risk of injury.

- Regular physical activity is crucial for physical health and mental peace.

- Exercise enhances energy, mood, and cognition, making it an effective tool for both body and mind.

- Exercise can be adapted to any fitness level, making it accessible to everyone regardless of age or ability.

Basic 101

The five primary types of exercises include:

- **Aerobic:** This type of exercise gets your heart rate up and increases your breathing. It improves your cardiovascular health, endurance, and overall fitness. Examples include brisk walking, running, swimming, cycling, dancing, and jumping rope.

- **Strength/Resistance:** This type of exercise builds muscle and strength. It can help you improve your posture, increase your metabolism, and reduce your risk of injury. Examples include weightlifting, bodyweight exercises, and resistance band training.

- **Flexibility:** This type of exercise improves your range of motion and flexibility. It can help you reduce muscle tension, improve your posture, and prevent injuries. Examples include yoga, tai chi, and stretching.

- **Balance:** This type of exercise improves your balance and coordination. It can help you reduce your risk of falls and improve your overall physical function. Examples include tai chi, yoga, and balance exercises on one leg.

- **Endurance:** This type of exercise improves your stamina and ability to sustain physical activity for extended periods. It can help you improve your cardiovascular health, muscle strength, and overall fitness. Examples include running, cycling, swimming, and hiking.

Actions

- Set both short-term and long-term fitness goals.

- Start with simple exercises and gradually increase intensity.

- Invest in quality exercise equipment and wear comfortable gear.

- Focus on sustainability—choose exercises that you truly enjoy and can maintain in the long run.

- Find a workout buddy or group for accountability and support.

- Schedule dedicated time for exercise in your daily routine.

Exercise Safely and Then Progressive Overload

Before starting any new exercise program, it's crucial to prioritize safety. This means understanding proper form and technique, listening to your body's signals, and gradually increasing intensity over time. Progressive overload is a key principle of exercise that involves gradually increasing the demands placed on your body to stimulate continued progress. This can be achieved by increasing weight, repetitions, sets, or the frequency of your workouts. However, it's essential to implement progressive overload safely to avoid injuries.

Here are some key points to remember:

- **Start with Proper Form and Technique:** Before adding weight or intensity, ensure you're performing exercises with the correct form to prevent injuries.

- **Listen to Your Body:** Pay attention to your body's signals and rest when needed. Pain is a warning sign that should not be ignored.

- **Warm Up and Cool Down:** Always include a warm-up before your workout and a cool-down afterward to prepare your body and prevent injuries.

- **Progress Gradually:** Gradually increase the duration, frequency, or intensity of your workouts over time. Avoid making drastic changes that could lead to burnout or injury.

- **Use Proper Equipment and Gear:** Wear appropriate clothing and footwear for your chosen activity and use safe, well-maintained equipment.

- **Consider Professional Guidance:** If you're new to exercise or have specific health concerns, consult with a qualified professional for personalized guidance.

- **Rest and Recovery:** Allow your body time to rest and recover between workouts to prevent overtraining and optimize results.

- **Stay Hydrated:** Drink plenty of water before, during, and after your workouts to stay hydrated.

- **Nutrition and Sleep:** Support your exercise routine with proper nutrition and adequate sleep for optimal recovery and results.

Element 3: Proper Daily Activities

How you spend your day plays a pivotal role in your overall health. By integrating movement and balance throughout your daily routine, you can maintain a dynamic and active lifestyle that supports weight loss and well-being.

Principles of Proper Daily Activities

- Avoid long periods of inactivity—frequent movement is essential for good health. You can use your phone timer or smartwatch to set sedentary warnings or movement reminders.

- Address unhealthy habits, such as smoking or excessive alcohol consumption, which can hinder progress.

- Incorporate physical activity into your daily routine, even in small ways. For example, parking further away, walking around while taking calls, or taking stairs instead of the elevator.

- Choose active hobbies and leisure activities that you enjoy.

- Prioritize getting enough sleep each night to support overall health and weight management.

- Manage stress effectively through relaxation techniques, mindfulness practices, and self-care.

- Foster social connections and engage in meaningful relationships that promote well-being.

- Find a balance between work, rest, and play to avoid burnout and maintain energy levels.

Basic 101

Daily activities encompass:

- **Sleep:** Aim for 7-8 hours of quality sleep to allow your body to rest and recover.

- **Work, Hobbies, and Social Interactions:** Engaging in activities that stimulate both your body and mind promotes overall well-being.

- **Relaxation:** Practices like meditation, yoga, or simply taking time for yourself can alleviate stress and promote mental health.

- **Active Transportation:** Choosing walking or cycling over driving for short distances increases daily movement and can contribute to weight loss.

- **Household Chores:** Activities like cleaning, gardening, and DIY projects can be surprisingly active and contribute to calorie expenditure.

- **Leisure Time:** Engaging in active leisure pursuits, like dancing, sports, or hiking, adds enjoyment and movement to your life.

- **Mindful Breaks:** Incorporating short breaks throughout the day for mindful breathing or stretching can help reduce stress and improve focus.

Actions

- Plan your day to ensure a balance of work, physical activity, and rest.

- Incorporate light movement throughout the day—whether through walking, gardening, or housework.

- Make time for self-care and relaxation to recharge and reduce stress.

- Take breaks throughout your workday to stretch, walk or do light exercises.

- Stand up and move around every 20-30 minutes if you have a desk job.

- Use active modes of transportation, like biking or walking.

- Schedule active leisure activities, such as dancing or playing sports.

- Prioritize sleep and rest to allow your body to recharge.

- Practice relaxation techniques, such as meditation or deep breathing.

- Connect with loved ones and engage in hobbies that bring you joy.

Element 4: Proper Food Supplements

Supplements can enhance the nutritional quality of your diet by filling in gaps and providing essential nutrients that may be lacking due to factors like limited food choices, medical conditions, or increased nutrient needs. However, it's important to remember that supplements should never replace whole foods. Instead, they should serve as a complementary tool to support your overall health. Whole foods offer a broader spectrum of nutrients and additional health benefits that supplements cannot replicate. Always prioritize a balanced, nutrient-dense diet, and consult with a healthcare professional before adding any supplements to your routine to ensure they are safe and suitable for your individual needs.

Principles of Proper Food Supplements

- **Supplements as Support, Not Substitutes:** Dietary supplements can be valuable tools for targeting specific nutritional deficiencies or supporting particular health goals. However, it's crucial to remember that they are designed to complement a well-rounded diet, not replace it. A balanced and diverse dietary pattern that includes a variety of whole foods remains the foundation of optimal health.

- **Personalized Supplementation:** The choice of supplements should be individualized and based on a comprehensive assessment of your unique health needs and dietary gaps. Factors to consider include your age, gender, activity level, medical conditions, current dietary intake, and any specific nutritional deficiencies identified through blood tests or other diagnostic assessments. Consulting with a registered dietitian or healthcare professional can be beneficial in determining the most appropriate supplements for your individual needs.

- **Quality and Safety:** Prioritize high-quality supplements from reputable manufacturers that adhere to Good Manufacturing Practices (GMP). Look for third-party certifications that verify the purity, potency, and safety of the product. Be cautious of exaggerated claims and potential interactions with medications or other supplements.

- **Dosage and Duration:** Follow the recommended dosage guidelines provided on the supplement label or as advised by your healthcare professional. Exceeding the recommended dosage can lead to adverse effects. Some supplements may be intended for short-term use to address specific deficiencies, while others may be beneficial for long-term maintenance.

- **Regular Monitoring and Evaluation:** Regularly reassess your supplement regimen and monitor its effectiveness in conjunction with your healthcare professional. Your nutritional needs and health status can change over time, and adjustments to your supplement plan may be necessary.

Basic 101

Common supplements include:

- **Omega-3 fatty acids:** Essential fats that our bodies cannot produce, so we must obtain them from diet or supplements. They offer numerous benefits, including supporting heart health, brain function, and reducing inflammation.

- **Probiotics:** Introduce beneficial bacteria (probiotics) into your gut, aiding digestion and overall health.

- **Herbal remedies:** Aloe vera and Tongkat Ali may offer benefits for digestion and stress relief.

- **Vitamin D:** Supports bone health, immune function, and mood regulation.

- **Multivitamins:** Provide a broad spectrum of essential vitamins and minerals.

- **Magnesium:** Plays a role in muscle function, nerve transmission, and blood sugar control.

- **Iron:** Essential for red blood cell production and oxygen transport.

- **Calcium:** Crucial for bone health and muscle function.

- **Protein:** Essential for building and repairing tissues, and supporting immune function. Supplemental protein is taken by those with higher daily protein requirements such as physically active individuals or those working out.

- **Vitamin C:** An antioxidant that helps boost immunity, aids in collagen synthesis, and supports overall health.

- **B Vitamins:** Essential for energy production, metabolism, and nervous system function.

- **Zinc:** Supports immune function, wound healing, and cell growth.

- **Creatine:** Can improve exercise performance and muscle strength. Besides that, creatine has also been shown to have cognitive benefits such as improving short-term memory and reasoning.

- **Glucosamine and Chondroitin:** Often used for joint health and to manage osteoarthritis symptoms.

- **Fiber Supplements:** Can aid in digestion, regularity, and weight management.

Actions

- Research any supplement you plan to take to ensure it has proven benefits. Consult with a healthcare professional or registered dietitian to determine if a supplement is necessary and safe for you.

- Prioritize whole foods for your nutrition and use supplements to enhance your diet.

- Choose supplements from reputable brands that have undergone third-party testing for quality and purity.

- Do not exceed recommended dosage, be aware of potential side effects and interactions with medications.

- Monitor your body's response to the supplement and adjust your intake as needed.

Element 5: Proper Monitoring

Regular monitoring of your health metrics ensures that you stay on track with your wellness goals. By tracking your progress, you can make adjustments and maintain motivation on your weight loss journey.

Principles of Proper Monitoring

- Monitoring your health metrics is essential to staying accountable.

- Key metrics to track include nutrition, physical activity, sleep, and mental well-being.

- Consistent tracking helps identify patterns and trends in your health data.

- Regular monitoring allows you to measure progress and celebrate achievements.

- Tracking your metrics provides insights that can guide adjustments to your diet and exercise routines.

- Monitoring helps you identify potential health issues early on.

Basic 101

What can be tracked?

1. **Physical Health**

   - Weight:

     o Body weight or body composition (weekly or bi-weekly)

     o Body fat percentage (monthly)

     o Waist circumference (monthly)

*Note: Regular weight monitoring, such as daily or weekly, can be stressful for some individuals. It's crucial to remember that weight isn't the sole indicator of overall health progress. Other aspects, like energy levels, sleep quality, and bloodwork, can show improvement even if weight remains static. Proper monitoring encompasses all health aspects, not just body weight. Avoid obsessing over the numbers on the scale, as it can lead to unnecessary stress.

- **Activity:**
  - Steps taken (daily)
  - Exercise duration and intensity (per workout)
  - Active minutes per day
- **Sleep:**
  - Hours of sleep per night
  - Sleep quality (using a sleep tracker or journal)
  - Time spent in different sleep stages (if using a sleep tracker)
- **Nutrition:**
  - Daily calorie intake
  - Macronutrient breakdown (protein, carbohydrates, fats)
  - Micronutrient intake (vitamins and minerals)
  - Hydration: Water intake
- **Bloodwork:** (consult with your doctor for frequency)
  - Cholesterol levels (total, HDL, LDL)
  - Blood sugar levels (fasting glucose, HbA1c)
  - Blood pressure
  - Thyroid function
  - Vitamin and mineral levels

2. **Mental Health**

   • **Mood:**

     o Daily mood ratings (using a mood tracker or journal)

     o Identify mood triggers and patterns

   • **Stress levels:**

     o Track daily stressors

     o Monitor physiological signs of stress (e.g., heart rate variability)

   • **Mindfulness & Relaxation:**

     o Time spent meditating or practicing mindfulness

     o Engagement in relaxing activities (e.g., reading, spending time in nature)

   • **Therapy/Counseling:**

     o Frequency of sessions

     o Progress towards therapeutic goals

3. **Relationships**

   • **Quality time:**

     o Time spent with loved ones

     o Meaningful conversations and shared activities

   • **Communication:**

     o Track instances of open and honest communication

     o Note any communication challenges

- **Social connections:**
  - Frequency of social interactions
  - Number of close relationships
  - Participation in social events

4. **Personal Growth**

- **Goal progress:**
  - Track progress towards personal goals (e.g., career, education, hobbies)
  - Break down larger goals into smaller, measurable steps

- **Skill development:**
  - Track time spent learning new skills
  - Monitor progress in acquiring new knowledge

- **Self-reflection:**
  - Journaling or regular self-reflection practices
  - Track personal insights and areas for growth

Actions

- Use fitness trackers or apps to monitor physical activity and sleep.

- Track your food intake to stay aligned with your nutrition goals.

- Regularly check in with how you're feeling mentally and emotionally.

- Take progress photos to visualize your physical changes over time.

- Measure your body composition (body fat percentage, muscle mass) periodically.

- Get regular medical checkups and blood tests to monitor your overall health and identify any potential issues.

- Seek support from a healthcare professional, registered dietitian, or certified trainer to interpret your health metrics and provide guidance.

Element 6: Positive Mental Attitude & Universal Success Principles

A positive mental attitude is a critical factor in achieving success. Embracing resilience and adopting principles from leading self-help experts can help you navigate challenges and stay focused on your goals.

Principles of Positive Mental Attitude

- Develop a clear vision for your life and goals.

- Build resilience to overcome obstacles and stay focused on your weight loss journey.

Basic 101

- **Vision**: Understand your purpose and why you want to achieve your goals.

- **Mission**: Define your goals and align them with your values.

- **Habits**: Establish good habits that reinforce success.

- **Resilience**: Strengthen your mental fortitude to handle setbacks.

Actions

- Take responsibility for your health and make decisions that align with your goals.

- Cultivate positive habits and learn from each experience.

Element 7: Personal Safety Culture

Safety is essential to every aspect of your life. By fostering a personal safety culture, you reduce the risk of accidents and create a more secure environment in which to thrive.

Principles of Personal Safety

- Personal safety is your responsibility. Set high safety standards for yourself.

- Cultivate a positive safety attitude to ensure you avoid unsafe actions at home, at work, and in the surrounding environment.

- Gain the knowledge and skills needed to identify and address safety hazards, unsafe conditions, and unsafe actions in all environments—whether at home, at work, or outdoors.

- Understand risk management concepts such as HIRAC (Hazard Identification, Risk Assessment, and Control) and the distinction between acceptable and unacceptable risks in accident prevention.

- Remember the formula: Risk = Probability × Severity.

- Take proactive steps to identify and eliminate hazards in your environment.

- Be aware of the risks involved in various activities and take appropriate measures to mitigate them.

Basic 101

In addition to being healthy and successful, it is crucial to develop a strong personal safety culture to minimize the risk of accidents and injuries in our daily lives. Unfortunately, many healthy and successful individuals suffer serious injuries or even die due to preventable accidents at home, during leisure activities, in the workplace, or on the road.

The risk of accidents can be significantly reduced by cultivating a personal safety culture. This involves taking proactive steps such as practicing defensive driving, identifying potential hazards in our environment, and taking action to eliminate those hazards. Setting high safety standards for ourselves and exercising self-discipline—such as always wearing a seatbelt, avoiding running red lights, and practicing other safety measures—can further reduce the risk of accidents.

Here are some essential safety topics to explore in order to build a strong safety foundation:

- Hazard Identification

- Electrical Safety

- Mechanical Safety

- Chemical Safety

- Use of Personal Protective Equipment (PPE) where necessary

- Traffic and Road Safety

- Fire and Explosion Safety

- Falls Prevention

- Noise Safety

- Ergonomics

- Construction Safety

- Safety and Health Laws

- Traffic Laws

Actions

- Continuously assess your environment for potential risks and take appropriate action to address them.

- Lead by example, fostering a safety-conscious culture within your home and community.

- Develop a strong interest in understanding safety and health topics.

- Actively participate in safety and health programs in the workplace or community.

- Attend safety and health courses to expand your knowledge.

- Learn from near misses and injury cases, and implement corrective and preventive actions to avoid similar incidents in the future.

Element 8: Personal Safety Plan

A Personal Safety Plan ensures that you are continuously prepared to avoid accidents and risks. Integrating this mindset into your daily routine allows you to lead a life that supports both physical and mental well-being.

Principles of Personal Safety Plan

- Prioritize safety in all aspects of your life, from your home to your workplace.

- Address unsafe behaviors and encourage proactive safety measures.

- Practice the mindset that "Safety is my No.1 Priority" in all daily activities.

- Embrace the Behavioral Safety Concept, focusing on safe attitudes, avoiding at-risk behaviors, and fostering safety leadership.

- Understand the root causes of unsafe behavior, such as urgency, taking shortcuts, lack of knowledge, poor housekeeping, and others.

- Develop a Personal Safety Plan as part of your overall Purpose, Vision, Mission, and Goals.

Basic 101

- Set clear safety goals that align with your broader wellness mission.

- Focus on behaviors that promote safer outcomes and mitigate risks.

- Maintain high safety performance standards.

- Implement behavioral safety practices.

- Develop safety habits through consistent, repetitive safe actions.

- Understand Risk/Hazard Identification, Risk Assessment, and Control (HIRAC), as well as the distinction between acceptable and unacceptable risks in accident prevention.

- Recognize and address safety hazards.

- Prevent accidents through lessons learned, root cause analysis, and corrective & preventive actions to avoid recurrence.

Actions

- Start now by embracing the motto: "Health & Safety is my No.1 Priority."

- Set both long-term and short-term health and safety goals as part of your PDCA (Plan-Do-Check-Act) cycle.

- Practice "Safety Leadership by Example" within your family.

- Conduct safety observations to identify unsafe acts and conditions in your home, car, home equipment, and surrounding areas, and take corrective actions to eliminate them.

- Regularly review and adjust your personal safety plan.

- Incorporate safety measures into your daily activities, ensuring your environment is conducive to health and well-being.

By embracing these 8 Key Elements of Healthy Living, you create a holistic approach to health that nurtures your body, mind, and environment. Together, these elements work synergistically to support not only your weight loss goals but also your long-term well-being. By focusing on these essential aspects of your life, you'll cultivate habits that lead to a balanced and fulfilling lifestyle, one that promotes health & safety, vitality, and sustained success.

Conclusion

In this chapter, we've explored the 8 Essential Elements of Healthy Living that provide a balanced foundation for sustainable weight loss and overall well-being. From proper nutrition and exercise to cultivating a positive mindset and ensuring personal safety, each element plays a crucial role in achieving long-term health goals. Remember, it's not about quick fixes or drastic changes—true transformation comes from adopting these elements as part of your daily routine and aligning them with your lifestyle. By focusing on each of these aspects, you create a holistic approach that supports your body, mind, and environment, setting the stage for lasting success.

Now that you have a deeper understanding of the fundamental elements of healthy living, it's time to turn that knowledge into action. The next chapter will guide you through the 6-Step Cycle for Continuous Improvement in Weight Loss, helping you integrate these principles into a dynamic process of growth, reflection, and progress. It's not just about losing weight, it's about building sustainable habits that will keep you on track, refine your approach, and help you achieve your goals with confidence. Let's dive into the next step of your journey!

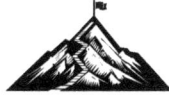

CHAPTER 5:

The 6-Step System for Continuous Improvement in Weight Loss

*"Today is your day, your mountain is waiting.
So.... get on your way."*

— Dr Seuss

n this chapter, we will share the 6 Steps to Fail-Proof, Sustainable Weight Loss and a Healthy Lifestyle, and explore the importance of using a SWOT analysis to evaluate your progress through a holistic system, including:

- Step 1: Easy Start: The Power of Caloric Deficit and Mastering the 8 Essential Elements of Healthy Living

- Step 2: Life Priorities and Alignment of Mind, Body, and Consciousness

- Step 3: A Systematic and Holistic Fail-Proof Plan-Do-Check-Act (PDCA) Continuous Improvement Cycle

- Step 4: Evaluating Progress with a Strengths, Weaknesses, Opportunities, and Threats (SWOT) Review

- Step 5: Refining the Health Plan

- Step 6: Iterative PDCA Continuous Improvement

These 6 steps are multifaceted, tailored approaches that empower and energize you to achieve long-term, sustainable healthy living with confidence.

We will dive deeper into how to apply these strategies in real life and translate these ideas into actionable steps that bring lasting change. This chapter will also provide practical examples, tips, and strategies for implementing the cycle and overcoming any obstacles along the way.

The 6-Step Cycle for Continuous Improvement is a flexible system that can be applied to all aspects of your weight loss journey and overall health. Each step builds on the previous one, keeping you focused and adaptable.

By the end of this chapter, you'll have a clear understanding of how to apply these tools to your daily routine. You will also be equipped with the resources needed to maintain progress and make steady improvements.

Diagram 5: 6 STEPS CONTINUOUS IMPROVEMENT CYCLE

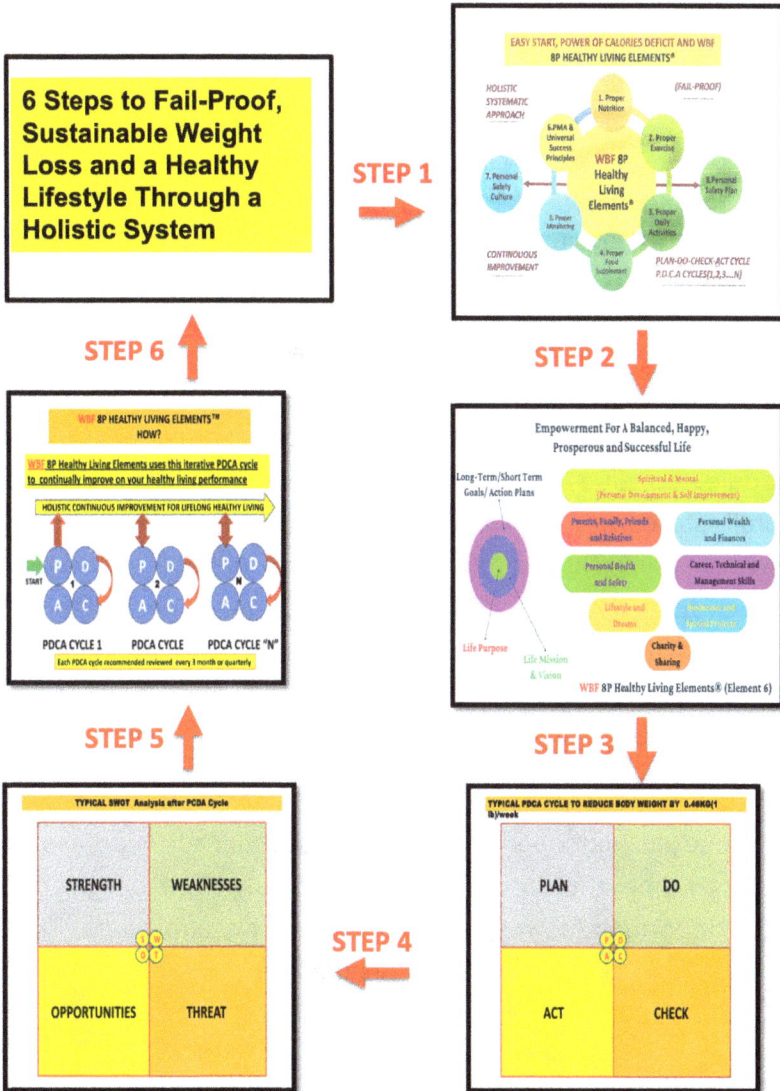

Step 1 & 2 can be illustrated as a plane taxiing from the parking bay to the runway before takeoff. Similarly, when conquering a mountain, these steps are like the preparatory work—such as acquiring proper knowledge and training, ensuring you have the right food and equipment, acclimatizing to the right attitude, mental preparation, and planning your routes—before setting out.

Step 3 is the takeoff of the plane or the beginning of the climb. As the plane takes off, the pilots must monitor the progress, ensuring that the plane climbs at the correct speed and angle to reach cruising altitude. Similarly, when starting the climb, you must monitor the route, watch for potential dangers, and stay alert to any obstacles along the way.

As shown in Diagram 6 on page 117, the unfortunate process of a person becoming obese typically takes place over many years, influenced by poor eating habits, a sedentary lifestyle, a busy schedule (no time for exercise), and stressful work. The body naturally stores visceral and subcutaneous fats as "reserve energy," a mechanism designed for survival during periods of famine or hunger. Unfortunately, our human bodies have not evolved to keep pace with the tremendous technological advances in society over the past few hundred years. This mismatch between our evolutionary biology and modern society, which was discussed earlier, contributes to the obesity crisis.

To reverse and conquer obesity, it is essential to recognize that it requires time and careful action. The body must be given the proper opportunity to respond to the fat removal process. This is why quick fixes and fad diets are unsustainable and ultimately fail.

Diagram 6: Journey to Obesity and Journey back to Normal/Lean

Poor eating habits, sedentary lifestyle, lack of sleep, poor habits low priority on health, stressful work – no time for exercise, many failed attempts- given up, lack of knowledge , lack of motivation,

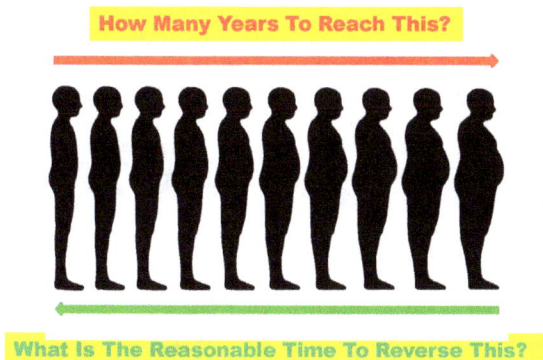

Good eating habits, active lifestyle, sufficient sleep, good habits, high priority on health, de-stressing activities. Allocate time for exercise, systematic and holistic approach, increase your knowledge , increasing motivation,

The 6 Steps to Fail-Proof, Sustainable Weight Loss and a Healthy Lifestyle through a Holistic System take into account the body's natural response time. Weight loss and healthy living are lifelong journeys, not a destination.

Achieving long-term, sustainable weight loss requires more than just following a diet plan or sticking to a temporary workout routine. True transformation involves adopting a strategic, holistic approach—one that continuously evolves through learning, adjusting, and improving. The 6-Step Cycle for Continuous Improvement in Weight Loss introduces a systematic, adaptable method that empowers you to take charge of your health and achieve lasting success. By integrating the Plan-Do-Check-Act (PDCA) cycle into your weight loss journey, you create a feedback loop that drives progress and helps you maintain momentum.

This chapter will walk you through each of these six steps, guiding you to master the essentials of healthy living, align your life priorities with your health goals, implement the PDCA cycle, evaluate your progress, refine your approach, and continue improving for sustainable results. Let's dive into how these steps will support you in creating lasting, transformative change.

Here's a breakdown of how to practically apply each step:

Step 1: Easy Start, The Power of Calorie Deficit, and Mastering the 8 Essential Elements of Healthy Living

Before diving into the PDCA cycle, it's crucial to first master the Easy Start, Power Of Calories Deficit and 8 Essential Elements of Healthy Living that form the foundation of your holistic health approach. These Easy Start, Power Of Calories Deficit and 8 Essential Elements lay the foundation for your weight loss journey and overall well-being. When you incorporate nutrition, exercise, sleep, mindset, safety, and the other elements into your lifestyle, you create a solid base for sustainable progress. These foundational habits are essential for success as they ensure you're not just focusing on weight loss, but on holistic health.Here's how you can practically integrate them into your daily routine:

- **Diet & Nutrition:** Plan your meals weekly. Include nutrient-dense foods like vegetables, fruits, lean proteins, and whole grains. A practical tip: start meal prepping on Sundays to ensure you have healthy meals ready throughout the week.

- **Exercise & Fitness:** Set realistic goals for physical activity, such as aiming for 30 minutes of walking, strength training, or yoga each day. Remember, consistency is key—even if you start with small bursts of activity.

- **Sleep**: Aim for 7-9 hours of restful sleep each night. Create a bedtime routine that includes winding down activities like reading or meditating.

- **Stress Management:** Incorporate daily relaxation techniques, such as deep breathing or mindfulness, to help reduce stress and enhance mental well-being.

Practical Example: Sarah, a busy professional, incorporates the 8 Essential Elements by starting her day with a 10-minute meditation session, preparing balanced lunches on Sundays, and ensuring she gets 8 hours of sleep. By following this, she sets herself up for success in all areas of her life.

Easy Start and the Power of Calorie Deficit is a baby step, a gentle, accessible approach for an obese or overweight person to begin their journey of conquering obesity and achieving lasting change. This step involves simple, stress-free physical activities, daily habits, and food adjustments that most people can incorporate into their lives without difficulty.

The key purpose of the Easy Start and Calorie Deficit approach is to help the individual develop a consistent, sustainable routine centered on nutrition, physical activity, and proper health monitoring. By focusing on small, manageable daily actions, significant weight loss can be achieved over time. Some practical steps include:

1. Brisk walking for 30 minutes and simple warm-up exercises such as stretching or bending for 15 minutes. This allows the individual to experience their body's response (e.g., sweating, body aches, increased energy) while enjoying fresh air and warm sunshine.

2. Reducing sugar in coffee and tea.

3. Eliminating sugary drinks.

4. Eating half portions of rice or starchy foods.

5. Cutting back on snacking.

6. Limiting or stopping alcohol consumption.

These small, consistent changes lay the foundation for long-term success, setting the individual on the path to sustainable weight loss and a healthier lifestyle.

The Easy Start approach, with its consistent and simple actions, is more sustainable and manageable for most busy individuals compared to intensive gym exercises, extreme diets, or high-intensity activities like marathon running. While such intense exercises are suitable for those who are already fit and exercise regularly, obese or overweight individuals should approach fitness cautiously and always consult their doctor before attempting any high-intensity workouts. Additionally, these intensive activities can be challenging for many working individuals who also have family responsibilities and demanding careers.

The Easy Start process should be followed for at least three months to build consistency and allow the person to understand how their body responds to exercise and dietary changes. During this time, it's important to learn to listen to the body and recognize when to stop during exercises. This awareness provides valuable data for the ongoing journey of sustainable weight loss and a healthy lifestyle.

Once the body becomes accustomed to the simple, consistent exercises and food control established during Easy Start, it's time to set more specific goals, introduce more structured and challenging physical activities, and refine calorie deficit control, health monitoring, and body-mind-consciousness alignment. At this stage, an obese or overweight person might begin with light walking (3,000 to 5,000 steps per day), controlling food portions by reducing carbohydrates and sugary drinks, cutting back on added sugars in coffee or tea, avoiding fatty fried foods, and drinking more water.

Step 1 also helps individuals gain a deeper understanding of their metabolism, eating habits, exercise patterns, and work-related stress. This gradual approach allows the person to slowly lean into the process, making lasting changes without feeling overwhelmed.

Step 2: Align Life Priorities and Mind-Body Balance

To achieve weight loss and maintain a healthy lifestyle, you must ensure that your health goals are in harmony with your larger life priorities. Mind-body alignment is key for both short-term weight loss and long-term health. If you neglect an aspect of your life—such as mental health, relationships, or career goals—it can create imbalances that affect your weight loss progress. Alignment between your personal priorities and mind-body balance is crucial to staying motivated and focused on your health goals.

Diagram 7: Empowerment For A Balanced, Happy, Safe, Healthy Prosperous and Successful Life

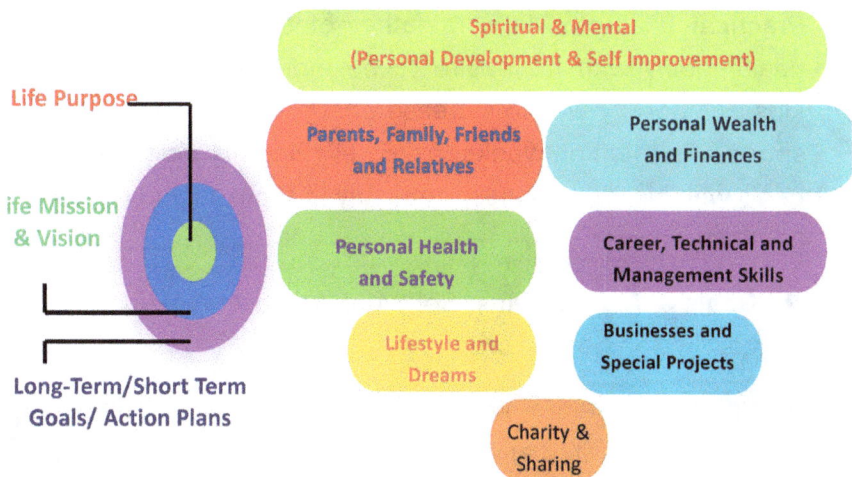

To align your life priorities effectively consider the following core areas:

- **Life Purpose, Vision & Mission:** Clarify what your life Purpose, Vision & Mission is beyond just weight loss. Do you want to be healthy to have more energy to play with your kids? To contribute more to society? To be healthy and successful in your career or business? To feel confident at a special event? Establish a deeper connection to your goal and Understanding why weight loss matters to you can deepen your commitment for your life that includes a healthy body and mind. Balancing on how different areas of your life—work, relationships, health—affect each other. If you're stressed at work, your health may suffer. Similarly, your social life could influence your eating habits or physical activity. Create a vision board that represents your life's priorities. Place it somewhere visible, like your office or bedroom, to keep you grounded in your purpose and remind you why weight loss is important for your bigger goals.

Practical Example: John, a father of three, aligned his health goals with his desire to be more active with his kids. His priority was to increase energy, so he could play sports with them on weekends. By aligning his weight loss goals with his life priorities, John stayed focused and made healthier choices.

- **Goals & Action Plans:** Set clear and actionable goals for your weight loss journey.

- **Spiritual & Mental Well-being:** Nurture your mental health to stay motivated and focused.

- **Personal Wealth and Finances:** Ensure your health goals are sustainable within your financial means.

- **Relationships (Family, Friends, Community):** Build supportive relationships that encourage your progress.

- **Career and Personal Growth:** Balance your weight loss goals with career ambitions.

- **Businesses and Special Projects:** Align your personal health goals with your business ventures.

- **Health and Safety:** Prioritize safety and injury prevention while pursuing fitness.

By recognizing that weight loss is only one piece of a much larger puzzle, an integral part of your other priorities can maintain balance in all areas of life. This approach helps prevent burnout, maintain motivation, and ensure that your journey toward a healthier life is sustainable.

Diagram 8 : ALIGNMENT OF MIND- BODY-CONSCIOUSNESS

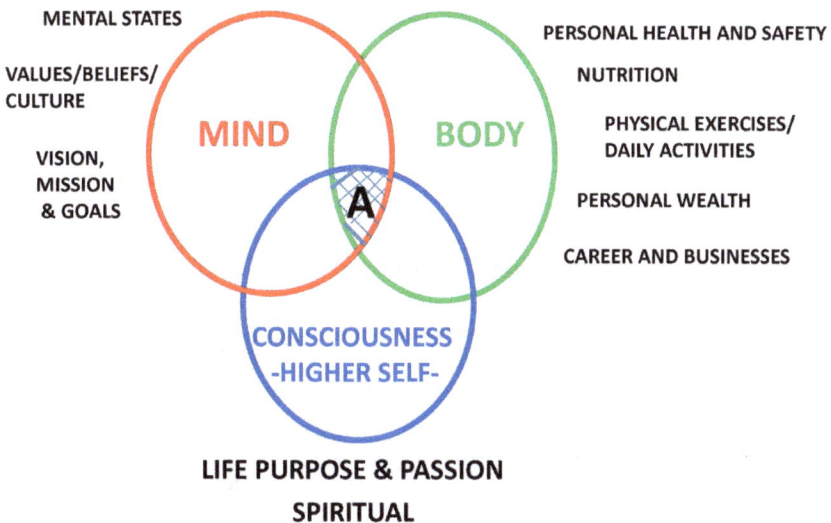

MENTAL STATES

VALUES/BELIEFS/
CULTURE

VISION,
MISSION
& GOALS

MIND

BODY

A

CONSCIOUSNESS
-HIGHER SELF-

PERSONAL HEALTH AND SAFETY

NUTRITION

PHYSICAL EXERCISES/
DAILY ACTIVITIES

PERSONAL WEALTH

CAREER AND BUSINESSES

LIFE PURPOSE & PASSION
SPIRITUAL

Alignment of Mind-Body-Consciousness fosters harmony in any actions or improvements you make towards better health, whether it's changing poor habits into healthy ones, such as losing weight, quitting smoking, or reducing excessive alcohol consumption. Never give up on your body—it's the only one you have. Love it, be kind to it, be tolerant of it, and always keep it clean, healthy, and safe.

Change can be difficult, uncomfortable, and sometimes emotional or painful, especially as you move out of your "comfort zone" toward the next level of growth. But remember, taking step-by-step actions, following the PDCA (Plan-Do-Check-Act) process, and making small achievements can lead to long-term sustainability. This gradual approach allows your mind-body-consciousness to adjust over time.

Your mind-body-consciousness is not a machine—it's an ancient, complex system that combines biological, chemical, mechanical, electrical, and electromagnetic processes with consciousness. Treat it with the patience and care it deserves as you move forward on your journey.

Step 3: Implement the First Plan-Do-Check-Act (PDCA) Cycle

The Plan-Do-Check-Act (PDCA) cycle as shown in Diagram 9 on page 126 is a proven method for continuous improvement that you can apply to every aspect of your weight loss journey. It helps you make informed decisions, assess progress, and refine your approach. Here's how you can implement the first PDCA cycle:

- **Plan:** Set clear, achievable 90-day weight loss goal. Identify key areas of your current routine that need improvement, such as adjusting your diet, increasing exercise intensity, or focusing on sleep. Establish a baseline and determine your action plan. For example, Sarah might plan to lose 6kg(14 pounds) in 90 days by reducing her daily calorie intake and increasing her exercise to 5 days per week.

- **Do:** Begin implementing small, manageable changes. For example, incorporate more vegetables into meals, reduce processed foods, or start walking more. Track your daily food intake, exercise routines, and how you feel physically and mentally.Take action by following the plan. For Example, Sarah starts tracking her calories using an app and commits to 45-minute workout sessions five days a week. She also drinks more water and increases her vegetable intake.

- **Check:** At regular intervals (such as weekly or bi-weekly), assess your progress. Are you on track to meet your goals? Are there any barriers hindering your success? This step helps you identify what is working and what needs adjustment. For example, after 4 weeks, Sarah checks her progress. She weighs herself and notices that she's lost 1 kg(2.2 pounds) instead of 2 kgs(4.4 pounds) as she is struggling with consistency on weekends and festive seasons..

- **Act:** Based on your evaluation, make necessary changes. If your initial approach isn't yielding results, adjust your diet, increase your workout intensity, or tweak your daily habits. Celebrate your small victories along the way to stay motivated. For example, Sarah tweaks her approach. She decides to meal prep on Saturdays and schedule 30-minute family walks in the evenings to stay active even on weekends and festive season.Another example, John's first PDCA cycle involved setting a goal to lose 2kgs (5 pounds) in 30 days. After reviewing his progress, he realized his biggest challenge was late-night snacking. To address this, he decided to incorporate a lighter dinner and a relaxing evening routine to avoid cravings.

Diagram 9: Plan-Do-Check-Act (PDCA)Cycle

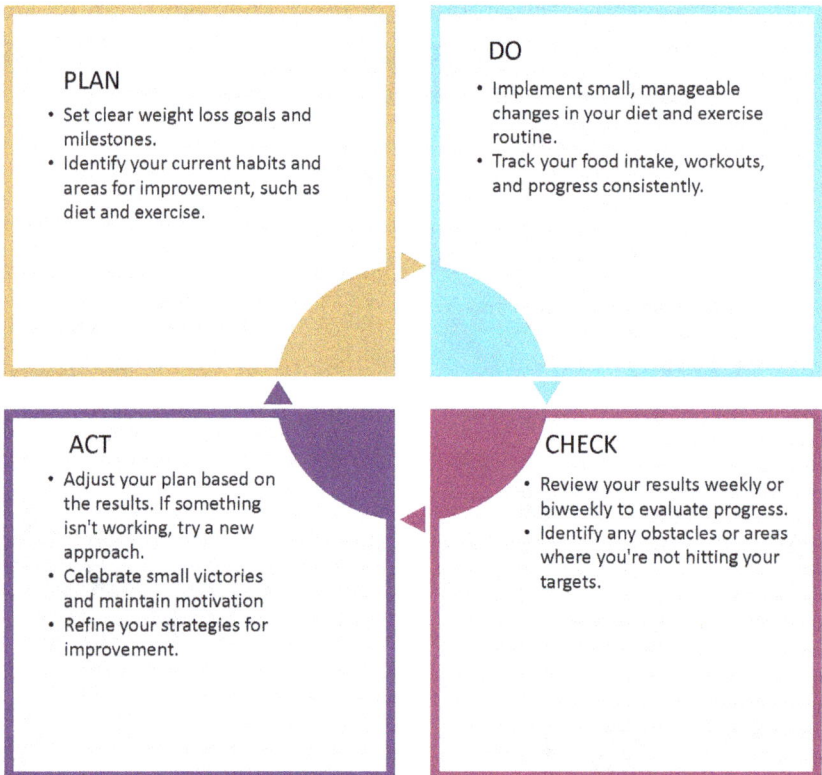

PLAN
- Set clear weight loss goals and milestones.
- Identify your current habits and areas for improvement, such as diet and exercise.

DO
- Implement small, manageable changes in your diet and exercise routine.
- Track your food intake, workouts, and progress consistently.

ACT
- Adjust your plan based on the results. If something isn't working, try a new approach.
- Celebrate small victories and maintain motivation
- Refine your strategies for improvement.

CHECK
- Review your results weekly or biweekly to evaluate progress.
- Identify any obstacles or areas where you're not hitting your targets.

The Iterative PDCA cycle as shown in Diagram 10 on page 127 isn't just about following a plan—it's about refining your approach regularly every 3 months to get better with each cycle after reviewing your Strength, Weaknesses, Opportunities and Threats(SWOT) review. This continuous improvement process allows you to achieve small results in a sustainable manner. These iterative cycles continue throughout your lifetime weight loss, weight maintenance and healthy lifestyle journey.

Diagram 10 : ITERATIVE PDCA CYCLES FOR CONTINUOUS IMPROVEMENT

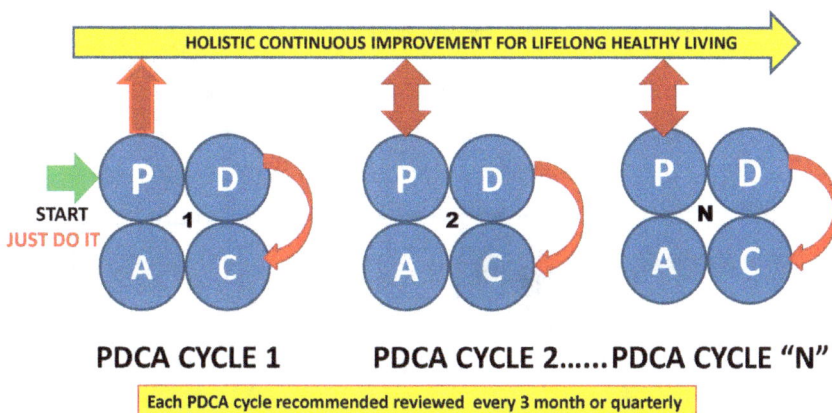

Step 4: Evaluate Progress with a SWOT Analysis

After completing the first PDCA cycle, it's time to reflect and evaluate your progress using a SWOT analysis as shown in Diagram 11 on page 128. This tool allows you to assess your internal and external factors, helping you understand where you can improve and where you're excelling.

- **Strengths:** What went well? Identify your successful habits and strategies.What positive changes have you made? Which habits or practices have you successfully incorporated into your routine during the first PDCA cycle?

- **Weaknesses:** Where did you struggle? Be honest and identify areas where you can improve? Are there any recurring challenges that need to be addressed, such as stress, lack of time, or emotional eating?

- **Opportunities:** What adjustments or new strategies can you implement to accelerate your progress? What new habits could enhance your progress? Are there tools, resources, or support systems you can leverage to improve?

- **Threats:** What external factors (stress, time constraints, social influences) could hinder or derail your progress? Are there environmental or situational stressors (like work deadlines or social pressures) that might affect your journey?

By honestly assessing these factors, you can identify areas for growth and take proactive steps to overcome obstacles.

Diagram 11: Strength Weaknesses Opportunities Threats(SWOT) Analysis

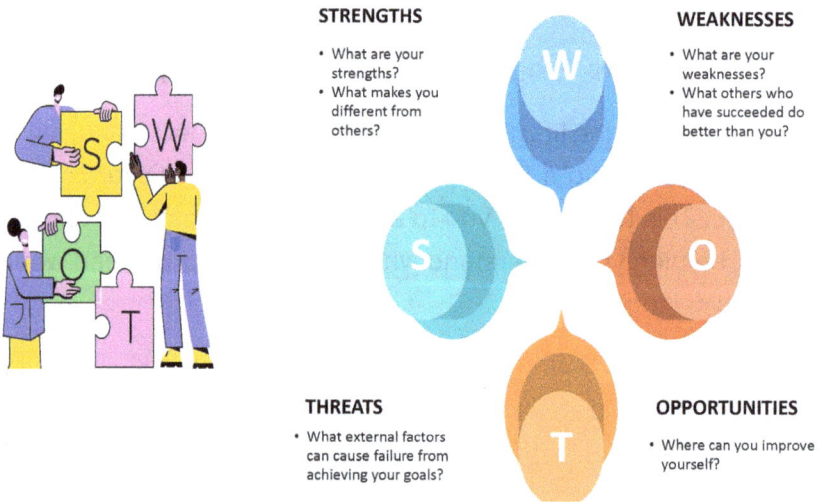

STRENGTHS
- What are your strengths?
- What makes you different from others?

WEAKNESSES
- What are your weaknesses?
- What others who have succeeded do better than you?

THREATS
- What external factors can cause failure from achieving your goals?

OPPORTUNITIES
- Where can you improve yourself?

Practical Example: Sarah did a SWOT analysis after completing her first PDCA cycle. She realized that her strength was meal prepping, but her weakness was her tendency to skip workouts on weekends. One opportunity she identified was taking a yoga class on Sundays, and a threat was her work schedule becoming unpredictable. She planned to schedule her workouts earlier in the week to prevent this issue. This will be incorporated in Sarah's second PDCA cycle in the next 3 months.

Step 5: Refine Your Healthy Living Plan

After conducting the SWOT analysis, use the insights to refine your healthy living plan and to adjust your goals, tweak your strategies, timeline and incorporate new habits that will help you stay on track. If certain areas are causing consistent challenges, explore new approaches to address them. This step is about evolving your plan based on what's working and what needs improvement.

This system promotes continuous improvement by achieving, recognizing, and celebrating small results over the course of 3 months (one PDCA cycle). It allows you to appreciate how far you've come in reaching those small milestones. For example, if your goal was to reduce the sugar in your coffee or tea from 2 teaspoons to none, and by the end of the 3-month PDCA cycle, you managed to consistently use just 1 teaspoon for 70 days, that's a huge achievement! The benefits to your health are significant—celebrate and pat yourself on the back!

This result proves that you can make changes and stick to them. Now, continue pushing to reach zero sugar in the next cycle. Afterward, conduct a SWOT analysis to review the lessons learned and apply the insights to the next cycle. Using the SWOT results from each PDCA cycle, focus on doing better in the next one. This iterative, repetitive process enables you to make gradual changes to your actions, habits, character, and ultimately, your culture and way of life.

With each cycle, you begin to understand and appreciate how your body responds to exercise, nutrition, food intake, and caloric consumption. This will strengthen your confidence, increase your passion and persistence, and fuel your motivation toward a healthier lifestyle.

By fine-tuning your approach, you make it more likely that you'll stay on track and continue seeing progress. Remember, this is an ongoing continuous process, and being flexible is key to long-term success. Conquering Obesity and Conquering Mountains is a journey not a destination. It involved step by step continuous improvement, celebrating small successes as you progress in your journey.

> **Practical Example**: John revised his plan after noticing that his weight loss had plateaued. He added more variety to his workouts, increased his water intake, and set a new goal to cut down on processed sugar. These adjustments helped him regain momentum.

Step 6: Repeat the PDCA Cycle for Long-Term Success

Weight loss and healthy living are not one-time efforts—they're lifelong commitments. To achieve lasting success, you must repeat the PDCA cycle as part of a continuous improvement process. Each time you cycle through these steps, you'll refine your approach, learn more about yourself, and grow stronger in your commitment to health and encourage you to stay flexible, adapt to new challenges, and celebrate small successes along the way. With each iteration, you'll build healthier habits, make sustainable progress, and achieve your ultimate goal of long-term weight loss and well-being.Over time, this will help you achieve long-term success in weight loss and health management.

> **Practical Example**: Sarah continues repeating the PDCA cycle, revising her plan each time based on her progress.

After six months, she's not only lost 9 kgs (20 pounds) but has also developed a sustainable, balanced lifestyle that she can maintain for life.

Maintaining Progress and Overcoming Obstacles

Even with a clear plan, obstacles will arise. The key is to stay focused and resilient. Here are some strategies for maintaining progress:

1. **Embrace Setbacks:** Understand that setbacks are a normal part of the process. When they happen, take a step back, reflect, and adjust your plan without losing motivation.

2. **Stay Accountable:** Find a support system, whether it's a workout buddy, a coach, or an online community. Sharing your progress and challenges can provide motivation and encouragement.

3. **Celebrate Small Wins:** Every milestone, no matter how small, deserves to be celebrated. This reinforces positive behavior and keeps you motivated.

4. **Keep Learning:** Continue to educate yourself about nutrition, fitness, and healthy living. The more you learn, the better equipped you'll be to refine your approach and overcome challenges.

Conclusion

By following the 6-Step Cycle for Continuous Improvement, you are embarking on a journey that goes beyond weight loss. You're committing to a holistic, sustainable lifestyle change that prioritizes your overall well-being. This approach ensures that every step you take is grounded in balance, reflection, and ongoing growth. As you move through each cycle, you'll refine your strategy, adjust your habits, and enhance your results, gradually building a life that not only supports your health goals but promotes your long-term success.

Remember, weight loss is not just about losing pounds, it's about creating lasting habits that improve all aspects of your life. The continuous improvement cycle empowers you to stay motivated, adapt to new challenges, and celebrate your victories, no matter how small. Each iteration of the cycle brings you closer to your ultimate goals, ensuring that your progress is not just measurable but sustainable. The beauty of this cycle is its adaptability. As life changes, so too can your goals and approach. This dynamic system ensures you're always evolving, improving, and reaching new milestones. You have the tools to make consistent, positive changes that will carry you through both the challenges and triumphs of your weight loss journey. Also, you'll not only experience physical transformation but also develop a mindset of continuous growth. The journey of weight loss and healthy living is a dynamic, ever-evolving process. Using the 6-Step Cycle builds the foundation for long-term success, ensuring that each day brings you closer to your health and wellness goals. The tools and techniques you've explored, including the SWOT analysis and PDCA cycles, provide a solid framework for sustainable growth in both weight loss and overall well-being. Always remember, the journey you're on isn't a quick fix, it's about making lasting changes that enhance every aspect of your life. Each PDCA cycle is an opportunity to refine your approach and move closer to your ultimate health goals. By staying committed to small, consistent improvements, you're setting yourself up for a lifestyle that not only supports your weight loss but also empowers you to thrive in every area of life.

This approach stands in stark contrast to quick-fix diets and instant gratification methods, which promise unsustainable results, much like cooking a bowl of instant noodles for a quick meal. There is a great deal of misinformation spread by irresponsible individuals looking to profit from the struggles of obese people, leading many to try various approaches based on false promises and hope. This results in many obese or overweight individuals giving up after repeated failures, often due to a lack of confidence.

For those seeking easy solutions or fast, linear weight loss results, consider this question: Why does it take 9 months for a woman to carry a baby and deliver it healthily? Most people naturally accept this timeline without hesitation because it's what we've been taught from a young age. No one would ever expect quick fixes, special exercises, or medications to deliver a healthy baby in just 5 months. Similarly, many obese or overweight people struggle to accept that the body needs sufficient time and sustained effort to lose weight in a natural, healthy way.

Just as it takes time to gain weight and become obese, it is equally important to understand that weight loss is a gradual process. You cannot become obese overnight, just as you cannot lose weight quickly through unsustainable methods. Both weight loss and pregnancy are natural biological processes that require time, effort, and patience.

As you continue applying the 6-Step Cycle, you will undoubtedly encounter challenges and obstacles, but with the strategies and insights you've gained, you'll be equipped to face them head-on. The key to success lies not just in your ability to adapt and refine your plans but in your commitment to building habits that support your long-term health and happiness.

In the next chapter, we'll dive deep into the psychology of habit formation and explore practical strategies for creating routines that support your health and wellness goals in the long term. Developing consistent, positive habits is the secret to maintaining progress, overcoming plateaus, and achieving sustainable success.

Now that you understand the power of the 6-Step Cycle and how it works as a framework for continuous improvement, it's time to dive deeper into how you can apply these principles to fine-tune your efforts and incorporate the 8 Essential Elements of Healthy Living into your daily life with greater clarity. Whether you're just starting or looking to refine your existing habits, this guide will equip you with the tools you need for continuous growth, helping you move closer to your goal of achieving sustainable health and wellness.

"You keep putting one foot in front of the other, and then one day you look back and you've climbed a mountain."

—Tom Hiddleston

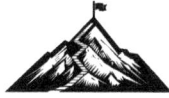

CHAPTER 6:

Building Habits That Stick

"The mountain is a metaphor for life; every climb is a chance to learn, grow, and become a better version of yourself."

—Unknown

Building lasting habits is the cornerstone of achieving long-term success in health and wellness. It's not enough to simply make temporary changes or follow fad diets that promise quick results. True, sustainable change is about creating new patterns of behavior that support your goals and become ingrained in your lifestyle. The road to this transformation is not always linear, and obstacles are inevitable. But with the right strategies, tools, and mindset, you can build habits that not only stick but become a natural and vital part of your everyday life.

Creating lasting habits requires patience, persistence, and a deep commitment to your health and well-being. It's about more than just achieving a particular goal—whether that's weight loss, improved fitness, or a healthier lifestyle. It's about shaping your daily routines in a way that aligns with your values and supports your long-term goals.

To successfully make these habits a permanent part of your life, you need to understand how to integrate them into your daily routine in a manageable and consistent way. The habits you build today will set the foundation for the person you become tomorrow. Whether it's waking up early to exercise, preparing healthy meals, or finding time to relax and recharge, small actions compound over time, leading to lasting, meaningful results.

In this chapter, we will explore actionable strategies for creating powerful habits that last. You will learn how to take small steps toward lasting change, using tools and techniques to stay accountable and motivated. You'll also discover how to manage setbacks and plateaus, which are inevitable parts of any journey, ensuring that you stay on track and continue progressing even when things get tough. By the end of this chapter, you'll have the insights and strategies to build habits that will propel you forward on your path to long-term health and wellness.

Creating Lasting Habits for Health and Wellness

Habits are the building blocks of our daily routines, and creating lasting habits is essential to achieving long-term success in your health journey. The good news is, with intention and the right strategies, you can form new habits that will support your weight loss goals and overall well-being.

1. **Start Small and Build Gradually**

   One of the biggest mistakes people make when trying to build new habits is overwhelming themselves with too many changes at once. Instead, start small. If you're looking to eat healthier, don't overhaul your entire diet in one go. Instead, try adding one vegetable to each meal or replacing one sugary snack with a healthier option. Once this becomes a routine, you can build on it by adding more changes over time.

2. **Make It a Daily Practice**

Consistency is the key to habit formation. Whether it's a 10-minute workout, preparing a healthy breakfast, or practicing mindfulness, incorporating your new habit into your daily routine is crucial. Make it non-negotiable, so it becomes a part of who you are. The more consistent you are, the more your habit will start to stick.

3. **Track Your Progress**

Tracking is essential to measure progress and to keep yourself accountable. Keep a journal or use a habit-tracking app to log your actions and celebrate small wins. When you can visually see your improvement, it boosts motivation and helps reinforce the habit. Plus, it helps you stay focused on your long-term goals.

4. **Pair New Habits with Existing Routines**

Pairing new habits with activities you already do regularly can make it easier to stick with them. For example, if you're trying to meditate, do it right after brushing your teeth in the morning. If you're aiming for a post-workout protein shake, prepare it as soon as you finish your exercise. This creates a natural flow and makes the new habit feel like a seamless part of your routine.

5. **Celebrate Your Wins**

Take time to celebrate your successes, no matter how small they may seem. Positive reinforcement helps to solidify habits and makes the process enjoyable. Treat yourself to something you enjoy when you complete a week of healthy eating or hit your workout goals. This keeps you motivated to keep going.

Tools for Staying Accountable and Motivated

Staying accountable and motivated is often the hardest part of building lasting habits. After the initial excitement wears off, it's easy to fall back into old patterns. Here are some tools to help you stay on track:

1. **Accountability Partners**

   Having someone to share your journey with can significantly increase your chances of success. This could be a workout buddy, a health coach, or even a friend who is also working toward similar goals. Regular check-ins help to keep you motivated and remind you that you're not alone in your journey.

2. **Set SMART Goals**

   Set **S**pecific, **M**easurable, **A**chievable, **R**elevant, and **T**ime-bound (SMART) goals for your habits. These types of goals provide clear direction and a way to measure progress. For example, instead of saying "I want to exercise more," say "I will exercise for 30 minutes, three times a week for the next month." This specific goal is easier to track and commit to.

3. **Visual Reminders**

   Set up visual cues to remind you of your new habits. If your goal is to drink more water, keep a water bottle on your desk or in your car. If you're focusing on stretching every day, place a yoga mat where you can easily see it. Visual reminders help trigger the behavior without needing to think about it actively.

4. **Create a Reward System**

   Rewarding yourself for reaching milestones reinforces the habit-building process. For instance, when you complete a full month of consistent workouts, treat yourself to a massage or a day off. These rewards should align with your goals—something that promotes health and wellness, rather than sabotaging your progress.

5. **Use Technology to Your Advantage**

   Apps can be powerful tools for staying accountable. From meal-planning apps to workout tracking apps, there are countless ways technology can support your habit-building journey. Some apps even offer social support features, where you can share your progress with others, helping to keep you accountable.

Overcoming Plateaus and Setbacks

No journey is without challenges. At some point, you may experience plateaus or setbacks, and it's important to be prepared for them. The key to overcoming these obstacles is maintaining a mindset of resilience and flexibility.

1. **Recognize That Plateaus Are Normal**

   Weight loss and personal growth don't always happen in a linear fashion. Plateaus are a natural part of the process. When your progress stalls, take a step back and assess your current habits. Are you pushing yourself too hard? Are there areas you can tweak or improve? Sometimes, a small change—like increasing your intensity or trying a new exercise—can help break through a plateau.

2. **Revisit Your Why**

   Remind yourself why you started this journey in the first place. Reflecting on your purpose and long-term goals can reignite your motivation. It's easy to get discouraged when progress slows down, but remembering your "why" can help you keep moving forward.

3. **Adjust Your Plan**

   If a setback occurs, don't see it as failure—view it as an opportunity to adjust and improve. Are there external factors that have contributed to your setback, such as stress, lack of sleep, or life changes? By identifying the root causes, you can modify your plan to make it more sustainable and realistic for your current situation.

4. **Stay Kind to Yourself**

   It's easy to be hard on yourself when setbacks happen, but self-compassion is key to long-term success. Mistakes are part of the process. Instead of criticizing yourself, practice self-kindness and focus on getting back on track, no matter how many times it takes.

5. **Keep the Big Picture in Mind**

   Don't lose sight of the fact that success is about consistency, not perfection. Progress may not always be fast, but every small step forward is still progress. Keep moving forward with patience and faith in your ability to succeed.

Conclusion

Building habits that stick is the cornerstone of long-term health and wellness. Achieving your health goals isn't about making dramatic changes overnight; it's about taking consistent, intentional steps that gradually add up to lasting, positive changes. As you move forward, starting small and being patient with yourself will help you create habits that integrate naturally into your daily routine, ultimately becoming the foundation of your healthier lifestyle.

Staying accountable and using the tools and strategies we've discussed in this chapter will guide you through any plateaus or setbacks you may encounter. No journey toward health and wellness is without challenges, but by maintaining a steady commitment to your habits and adapting as needed, you can build resilience and continue making progress. The power of habit lies in its ability to persist, even when motivation fluctuates. As your new habits become ingrained in your daily life, they will help you push through the inevitable obstacles that come your way.

The road to long-term success is not always easy, but the right mindset and effective strategies will keep you moving in the right direction. Achieving your health goals isn't just about reaching a specific target; it's about creating a lifestyle that supports your well-being for years to come. When you build habits that stick, you unlock the ability to sustain your progress, navigate challenges, and embrace each new chapter of your journey with confidence and purpose.

As you continue to apply the principles of habit-building in your own life, understand that each step you take brings you closer to the person you want to become. It's not about achieving perfection, but about consistency and progress. By embracing this approach, you're not only transforming your health, but you're also setting yourself up for a lifetime of wellness, empowerment, and fulfillment.

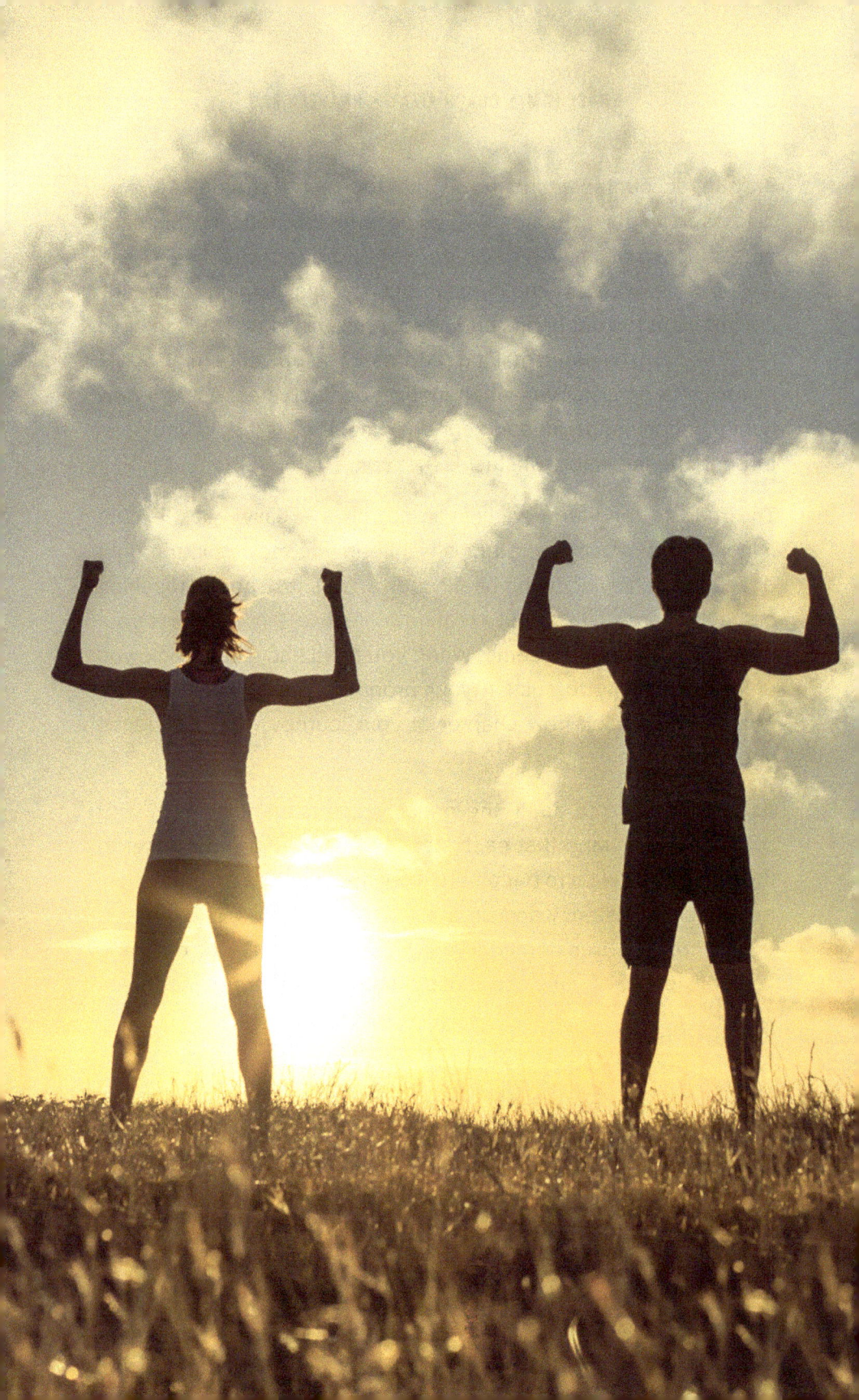

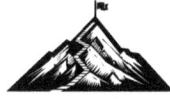

CHAPTER 7:

Achieving Success and Wellness Simultaneously

"Celebrate your success, but never forget the lessons learned along the way."

—Unknown

Defining Success and Wellness

uccess and wellness are two concepts that hold significant importance in our lives, especially for busy professionals seeking a truly fulfilling existence. In this chapter, we delve into the exploration of defining success and wellness for oneself, with the objective of creating a balanced life blueprint that aligns both elements harmoniously.

It is not uncommon for society to have preconceived notions of what success and wellness should look like. We are bombarded with external standards and expectations that often leave us feeling overwhelmed and disconnected from our true selves. However, the first step towards achieving genuine success and wellness lies in defining these concepts on our own terms.

To begin this journey, take a moment to ponder what success really means to you. Is it climbing the corporate ladder and achieving financial stability? Or does it encompass personal growth, relationships, and making a positive impact in the world? Success is a deeply personal concept, and by defining it for ourselves, we pave the way towards a more fulfilling life.

Similarly, wellness is not a one-size-fits-all concept. While physical health plays a significant role, wellness extends beyond the realm of mere exercise and nutrition. It encompasses mental, emotional, and spiritual well-being as well. Reflect on what truly makes you feel nourished and balanced in all aspects of your life. Is it practicing mindfulness, pursuing creative outlets, or cultivating meaningful connections? Dig deep into your core values and desires to establish a comprehensive definition of wellness peculiar to your unique self.

Once you have defined success and wellness individually, the next step is to integrate these aspects into a cohesive blueprint that promotes balance. Striving for success without considering wellness can leave us feeling burnt out and unfulfilled, while focusing solely on wellness may hinder our growth and limit our potential.

To achieve a balanced life blueprint, allow success and wellness to intertwine and complement each other. Create a vision that considers both elements coexisting harmoniously. What does it look like to be successful while maintaining your well-being? How can you pursue your professional ambitions without sacrificing vital aspects of your personal life? Find the intersection where success and wellness converge and thrive.

This is not about conforming to societal expectations but rather defining success and wellness in a way that aligns with your values, passions, and aspirations. Embrace the journey of introspection and self-discovery, for it will be the foundation upon which your balanced life blueprint is built.

Keep in mind that defining success and wellness is an ongoing process. It evolves with time and as you delve deeper into your personal growth. Embrace the flexibility to refine and redefine these concepts as you progress through life, always striving for a more harmonious balance.

Life Assessment: Evaluating Your Current State

As busy professionals, we are constantly striving for success and wellness in our lives. We juggle demanding careers, personal relationships, and self-care, all while trying to maintain a sense of balance. However, it can feel overwhelming at times, leaving us wondering if we are truly on the right path.

In order to achieve success and wellness simultaneously, it is crucial to take a step back and conduct a comprehensive life assessment. This assessment will allow us to identify areas in need of improvement and areas of strength, providing us with a roadmap towards a more balanced and fulfilling life.

The first step in conducting a life assessment is to take an honest inventory of our current state. This requires us to evaluate various aspects of our lives, including our physical health, mental well-being, relationships, and overall satisfaction. By examining each of these areas closely, we can gain valuable insights into what is working well and what areas require our attention.

When assessing physical health, it is essential to consider factors such as exercise, nutrition, and sleep. Ask yourself, "Am I dedicating enough time to physical activity? Is my diet nourishing my body? Am I getting enough restorative sleep?" Identifying areas where improvements can be made will allow you to develop healthier habits and enhance your overall well-being.

Next, delve into your mental well-being. Reflect on your thoughts, emotions, and overall mental outlook. Are you experiencing excessive stress or anxiety? Do you prioritize self-care and relaxation? Evaluating your mental state will help you identify areas where you can prioritize your mental health and incorporate practices such as mindfulness or therapy to foster a more positive mindset.

Relationships play a crucial role in our lives, and assessing the quality of our connections is essential. Consider the dynamics of your relationships with family, friends, and colleagues. Are these relationships supportive and fulfilling? Do you invest enough time and effort into nurturing these connections? Identifying areas where you may need to improve communication or establish stronger boundaries can lead to healthier and more fulfilling relationships.

You also need to evaluate your overall satisfaction and fulfillment in life. Reflect on your goals, aspirations, and values. Are you aligned with your authentic self? Do you feel a sense of purpose in your daily activities? It is vital to assess whether your current path aligns with your long-term vision and values, as this will guide your decisions and actions moving forward.

Conducting a comprehensive life assessment is the first step towards achieving success and wellness simultaneously. By identifying areas in need of improvement and areas of strength, you can create a blueprint for a more balanced and fulfilling life. Success and wellness are not static ideals but ongoing journeys that require continuous self-reflection and growth. Stay committed to your path, embrace the possibility of change, and take the necessary steps to align your actions with your goals and values.

Setting Meaningful Goals

Do you often find yourself overwhelmed, chasing after success while neglecting your overall well-being? Many busy professionals face this dilemma, striving to reach their professional ambitions but sacrificing their personal lives in the process. The key to achieving success and wellness simultaneously lies in setting meaningful goals that align with both sides of your life.

Setting goals is an art that requires careful consideration and planning. It goes beyond simply listing your desires; it involves crafting a blueprint for your life that supports and fosters both your career and your personal well-being. When done effectively, goal setting becomes a powerful tool for guiding your actions and ensuring that every step you take leads you closer to your ideal life.

The first step is to gain clarity on what success means to you. Take a moment to reflect on your professional ambitions and identify what truly drives you. Is it the pursuit of a prestigious position? Financial stability? Making a meaningful impact in your industry? Whatever it may be, remember that success is a subjective concept. It is essential to define it on your own terms, aligning it with your values and passions.

Equally important is understanding the significance of your personal well-being. Achieving success should not come at the cost of sacrificing your mental, emotional, and physical health.

If you neglect these aspects, the journey towards success may become an arduous one filled with burnout and dissatisfaction. Take the time to identify what brings you joy, what makes you feel alive, and what gives you a sense of fulfillment outside of your professional life.

Once you have gained clarity on both your professional ambitions and personal well-being, it is time to set meaningful goals. Effective goal setting requires you to be specific, measurable, achievable, relevant, and time-bound (SMART). By applying the SMART framework, you ensure that your goals are concrete and actionable.

Start by breaking down your long-term vision into bite-sized and manageable goals. Establish milestones that will guide your progress and give you a sense of accomplishment along the way. Remember to align these goals with both your professional and personal aspirations, allowing them to complement and support each other rather than compete.

Furthermore, it is crucial to make your goals resonate with your passions and values. When your goals are aligned with what truly matters to you, you will find the motivation and commitment required to stay focused and determined. This alignment between your goals and your passions will fuel your drive, making the journey towards success and wellness an exhilarating one.

One powerful strategy for setting meaningful goals is to visualize your desired outcome. Take a moment to imagine yourself living a life that encompasses both success and wellness. Close your eyes and picture the person you want to become, the achievements you aspire to, and the fulfillment you will experience in all aspects of your life. Immerse yourself in the emotions associated with this vision, allowing them to fuel your passion and drive. By consistently visualizing your goals, you create a powerful mindset that propels you forward, even when faced with obstacles.

Another crucial element in goal setting is breaking them down into smaller, actionable steps. As the saying goes, "Rome wasn't built in a day." Similarly, your path to success and wellness cannot be achieved in one giant leap. By breaking your goals into smaller milestones, you create a roadmap that guides your progress and keeps you motivated along the way. Celebrate each milestone achieved, as it signifies another step forward towards your ultimate destination.

It is inevitable that you will encounter roadblocks and setbacks on your journey. During these moments, it is essential to stay focused, determined, and resilient. Cultivate a growth mindset that sees challenges as opportunities for learning and growth rather than as insurmountable barriers. Embrace setbacks as valuable lessons that provide valuable insights into areas that may need adjustment or improvement. Remember, it is not the setbacks that define you but how you respond to them.

Throughout your journey, finding balance between your professional and personal pursuits will be crucial. Remember that achieving success and wellness simultaneously requires you to prioritize and allocate time and energy to both aspects of your life. Set boundaries and honor them, ensuring that you have dedicated periods for work, rest, and enjoyment. By establishing this harmony, you will find that you can excel in both domains without sacrificing one for the other.

Embrace the unknown, be open to new possibilities, and adapt your goals as necessary. This is your blueprint to a balanced life, crafted with your values and passions as the foundation.

Time Management: Maximizing Efficiency

As busy professionals pursuing a successful life, our days can often become overwhelming and chaotic. The constant demands on our time and attention can leave us feeling like we're being pulled in a million different directions. It's no wonder that many of us struggle to find a sense of balance and harmony in our lives.

But fear not, we will uncover techniques to effectively manage your time and increase productivity while maintaining that crucial balance. By implementing these strategies, you will be able to conquer your to-do list with ease and experience a greater sense of fulfillment in both your personal and professional life.

Let's kick things off by acknowledging the importance of prioritization. Too often, we find ourselves frantically trying to juggle an overwhelming number of tasks, without taking a moment to assess which ones truly deserve our attention. Setting clear goals and priorities is the first step towards effective time management. Take a moment to reflect on what matters most to you and align your tasks accordingly.

Another powerful technique to maximize efficiency is the art of delegation. It's easy to fall into the trap of wanting to do everything ourselves, believing that no one else can do it as well as we can. However, learning to delegate tasks to capable individuals not only lightens our workload but also empowers those around us. Remember, success is not about doing everything—it's about working smartly and effectively.

Next, let's explore the concept of time blocking. This technique involves breaking your day into specific blocks of time allocated for different activities. By assigning dedicated blocks for tasks like email correspondence, project work, and self-care, you create a structured schedule that allows for increased focus and productivity. Remember to also allow time for breaks and relaxation to recharge your mind and prevent burnout.

We live in a world filled with distractions—constant notifications, endless meetings, and the pressure to always be available. To achieve the balance we seek, it's crucial to establish boundaries around our time and energy. Learn to say no to tasks that don't align with your priorities, and create space for activities that truly bring you joy and fulfillment.

Now, let's dive even deeper into advanced strategies that will further enhance your time management skills and propel you towards success and wellness.

One powerful technique to boost your productivity is the Pomodoro Technique. This method involves breaking your work into 25-minute intervals, called Pomodoros, and taking short breaks in between. By working in focused bursts and incorporating frequent breaks, you can maintain high levels of concentration, prevent burnout, and maximize your efficiency. Set a timer for each Pomodoro, eliminate any potential distractions, and watch as your productivity soars.

Another advanced technique to explore is batch processing. This method involves grouping similar tasks together and dedicating a specific timeframe to complete them all at once. This eliminates the inefficiency of switching between different types of tasks and allows you to enter a state of flow. For example, instead of responding to emails throughout the day, set aside specific blocks of time to tackle all your email correspondence in one go. By doing this, you'll save time, improve focus, and gain a sense of accomplishment.

Furthermore, embracing technology can significantly streamline your time management efforts. There is a wide range of productivity tools and apps available that can help you organize your tasks, set reminders, and automate repetitive processes. Experiment with different tools to find the ones that work best for you, whether it's a project management software, a digital calendar, or a task-tracking app. Embracing these technological advancements will revolutionize your efficiency and leave you with more time to focus on what truly matters.

Lastly, occasional self-reflection is a valuable practice to incorporate into your time management routine. Take a moment to review your progress and analyze any areas where you can further enhance your efficiency. Celebrate your successes, acknowledge areas where you have improved, and make adjustments to areas that need refining. This self-reflection will keep you on track and motivated to continue your journey towards achieving success and wellness in balance.

By implementing these advanced techniques and strategies, you have unlocked the key to achieving optimal productivity without sacrificing your sense of balance and harmony. Time is a precious resource, and how you choose to spend it determines your success and well-being.

Nurturing a Supportive Network

In today's fast-paced world, it can be easy to get caught up in the hustle and bustle of our careers, striving for success and aiming for that elusive sense of achievement. We dedicate countless hours to our work, tirelessly pushing ourselves to climb the ladder of success. However, as we focus relentlessly on our professional endeavors, we often overlook the importance of nurturing a supportive network and fostering meaningful relationships.

Building a strong support network is not just a nice-to-have; it is an essential component of a well-rounded and fulfilling life. When we surround ourselves with people who uplift and inspire us, we create an environment that is conducive to both personal growth and professional success. These connections provide the foundation for a balanced and harmonious life, where our well-being and career thrive simultaneously.

One of the key benefits of nurturing a supportive network is the wealth of knowledge and experience it brings. By forging meaningful connections with individuals from various walks of life, we gain access to a diverse range of perspectives and insights. These interactions broaden our horizons, challenge our assumptions, and open doors to new opportunities we may have never considered. Whether it's seeking advice from a mentor or collaborating with like-minded professionals, a supportive network allows us to tap into a collective wisdom that propels our growth and development.

Moreover, a strong support network offers a reliable safety net during times of challenge and adversity. In the pursuit of success, we are bound to encounter obstacles and setbacks along the way. During these trying moments, having a network of supportive individuals who believe in our abilities and offer encouragement can make all the difference.

A supportive network not only bolsters our resilience but also provides emotional support. The importance of having someone to lean on during tough times cannot be overstated. Knowing that we have people who genuinely care about our well-being and are there to lend an empathetic ear or a helping hand can be immensely comforting. These relationships remind us that we are not alone in our journey and instill a sense of belonging that is essential for our overall well-being.

Additionally, a strong support network can have a profound impact on our professional lives. As we connect with individuals who have similar ambitions and goals, we find opportunities for collaboration, mentorship, and knowledge-sharing. The power of networking should not be underestimated, as it can lead to career advancements, strategic partnerships, and even new business ventures. By nurturing these relationships, we create a web of connections that not only enhance our current work but may also shape our future opportunities.

Building a strong support network and fostering meaningful relationships is crucial for both personal well-being and professional success. It provides us with diverse perspectives, emotional support, and opportunities for growth. As busy professionals pursuing a successful life, we must prioritize the cultivation of these connections, for they form the fabric of a balanced life blueprint.

The first step in building a strong support network is to identify the individuals who will uplift and inspire you on your journey. Seek out those who share your values, passions, and ambitions. Look for people who not only believe in your potential but also challenge you to push beyond your limits. These connections will provide the foundation for a supportive network that nurtures both your personal and professional growth.

Once you have identified potential individuals, it's essential to invest time and effort in cultivating these relationships. Start by reaching out and expressing your interest in connecting. Be genuine and show a sincere desire to learn from and support one another. Regularly engage in meaningful conversations, whether it's over a cup of coffee, a lunch meeting, or even a virtual chat. True connections are built through open and honest communication.

Networking is a two-way street. Show genuine interest in others' journeys and offer support and guidance whenever you can. By being a valuable resource and a trustworthy ally, you contribute to the growth of your network as well. Collaboration and mutual support lay the groundwork for long-lasting and fruitful relationships.

Another powerful strategy for nurturing a supportive network is actively participating in communities and associations related to your field or interests. Attend industry conferences, workshops, or meetups to connect with like-minded professionals who can offer unique perspectives and potential collaborations. Join online forums, LinkedIn groups, or social media communities where you can engage in discussions and share experiences with others who are passionate about similar topics.

When it comes to expanding your support network, don't limit yourself to individuals in your immediate circle. Embrace diversity and seek connections beyond your usual comfort zone. Step outside of your industry or field and explore opportunities to connect with individuals from different backgrounds, cultures, or areas of expertise. These varied perspectives can bring fresh insights and innovative ideas that you can apply to your own professional endeavors.

Lastly, always be open to new experiences and be willing to give back to your network. Offering guidance, mentorship, or support to others not only helps them grow but also deepens your own sense of purpose and fulfillment. In nurturing and expanding your support network, you impact not only your own success but also the success of those around you.

Building a strong support network requires genuine effort, constant engagement, and a willingness to step outside of your comfort zone. By nurturing connections that inspire and uplift you, you can create a supportive environment that fuels your personal and professional growth. Success and wellness are not mutually exclusive; they thrive when cultivated together through the power of supportive relationships.

Cherish the connections you have, foster new relationships, and never underestimate the power of a strong support system. With a well-nurtured network by your side, the possibilities for success and wellness are truly boundless.

Prioritizing Self-Care

In the hustle and bustle of today's fast-paced world, it's easy to get caught up in the never-ending cycle of work, appointments, and obligations. As busy professionals pursuing successful lives, we often neglect the most crucial aspect of our well-being: self-care. However, prioritizing self-care is not only essential for our overall health and happiness, but it is also a key ingredient for achieving sustained success.

Self-care goes beyond the occasional spa day or taking a break from work. It involves a holistic approach that encompasses our physical, mental, and emotional well-being. By investing time and energy into catering to these different aspects of ourselves, we can ensure we show up as the best version of ourselves in every aspect of our lives.

Physical self-care forms the foundation of our well-being. It involves nourishing our bodies through regular exercise, adequate sleep, and a balanced diet. Engaging in physical activities we enjoy releases endorphins, reducing stress levels and boosting our mood. Making space for regular exercise not only improves our physical health but also enhances our mental clarity, allowing us to tackle challenges with greater focus and creativity.

Mental self-care is equally vital in our pursuit of success and wellness. Our minds require regular nourishment and stimulation to thrive. Engaging in activities that challenge our intellect, such as reading, engaging in creative pursuits, or learning something new, helps expand our horizons and keeps our minds sharp. Taking time for reflection and relaxation through practices like meditation or journaling can promote mental clarity and reduce stress levels, leading to enhanced productivity and overall well-being.

Emotional self-care revolves around nurturing our emotional well-being. This aspect involves recognizing and addressing our emotions, seeking support when needed, and engaging in activities that bring us joy and fulfillment. Whether it's spending quality time with loved ones, pursuing hobbies, or practicing mindfulness, these actions can foster emotional resilience, improve our relationships, and contribute to our overall sense of happiness and contentment.

By prioritizing self-care, we create a solid foundation that supports our pursuit of success and wellness simultaneously. When we neglect ourselves, burnout and dissatisfaction become inevitable, hindering our ability to thrive in our personal and professional lives.

Imagine a life where we can comfortably juggle our career ambitions while still maintaining optimal well-being. Picture a world where success and self-care seamlessly coexist, each amplifying the other. It is not only possible, but it is within our grasp.

One effective strategy to incorporate self-care into your daily routine is by implementing effective time management techniques. Prioritize your well-being by scheduling dedicated time for activities that nourish your body, mind, and soul. Whether it's going for a morning jog, reading a few chapters of a book, or practicing mindfulness, make these self-care practices non-negotiable appointments with yourself. By treating self-care as a priority rather than an afterthought, you can ensure that you consistently nurture all aspects of your well-being.

It's equally important to cultivate a mindset of self-compassion and self-acceptance. As high-achieving professionals, we often place immense pressure on ourselves to meet unrealistic expectations. This mindset can lead to burnout and hinder our journey towards balanced success. So, remember to be kind to yourself, celebrate your accomplishments, and embrace imperfections as part of your growth process. By cultivating self-compassion, you can foster a healthier and more balanced approach to success.

Another valuable practice to prioritize self-care is setting boundaries. As professionals, we frequently push ourselves beyond our limits, taking on excessive commitments and overextending ourselves in the pursuit of success. However, establishing clear boundaries is crucial for preventing burnout and maintaining sustained well-being. Learn to say no when necessary and possess the courage to protect your time and energy. By doing so, you create space for self-care practices and ensure that you have the capacity to show up fully in all areas of your life.

Self-care does not have to be a solitary journey. Surround yourself with a support system of like-minded individuals who understand the importance of balancing success and wellness. Seek accountability partners who can hold you responsible for prioritizing self-care and provide support when challenges arise. Additionally, consider seeking professional guidance through coaching or therapy to gain valuable insights and tools to navigate the complexities of balancing success and well-being.

Lastly, embrace the power of gratitude and mindfulness. Cultivating a gratitude practice can shift your perspective and enhance your overall well-being. Take a few moments each day to reflect on the things you are grateful for, both big and small. Practicing mindfulness allows you to fully engage in the present moment, reducing stress and fostering a sense of calm. Incorporate simple mindfulness exercises such as deep breathing or mindful eating into your daily routine to enhance your self-care journey.

By implementing these practical tips and tricks, you are taking proactive steps towards achieving true success and wellness simultaneously. Self-care is not a luxury but a necessity for all who seek a fulfilling and balanced life. As a busy professional, you deserve to prioritize your well-being without compromising your ambitions. So, embrace the power of self-care, create a foundation of well-being, and watch as sustained success naturally unfolds in your life.

Conclusion

As we reach the end of this chapter, take a deep breath and carry with you the powerful realization that you already possess the key to achieving success and wellness in harmony. These two essential aspects of life are not mutually exclusive—they can coexist, complement one another, and create a foundation for a fulfilling and purposeful life.

The path to balance is rarely straightforward. It may present obstacles, moments of doubt, and unexpected turns. Growth often comes through challenge, and within every challenge lies an opportunity to rise stronger, wiser, and more aligned with your true self.

By choosing to prioritize self-care, you affirm that your well-being is not a luxury—it is a necessity. When you implement effective time management techniques, you reclaim control over your day and create space for what truly matters. By practicing self-compassion, you shift from self-judgment to self-acceptance, allowing yourself to move forward without the weight of unrealistic expectations.

Setting healthy boundaries gives you the strength to protect your time, energy, and emotional peace. Reaching out and seeking support connects you with others who uplift and understand you—reminding you that you're not alone on this journey. And by embracing gratitude and mindfulness, you learn to find joy in the present moment and develop a deeper appreciation for life, no matter how busy or demanding it becomes.

These practices are not quick fixes; they are lifelong tools—powerful habits that, when cultivated with intention, can transform the way you live, work, and thrive.

So, stay committed. Keep choosing yourself, your growth, and your wellness, even when the world pulls you in a hundred different directions. Know that every step you take toward balance is a step toward a more vibrant, energized, and successful version of yourself.

The journey to achieving success and wellness is not just about the destination—it's about who you become along the way. And the possibilities that lie ahead? They are nothing short of extraordinary.

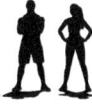

THE CONCLUSION: YOUR JOURNEY TO A HEALTHIER LIFE

"The summit is the goal, but the camaraderie, the challenge, the sheer joy of movement—that's the heart of the climb."

—Unknown

As you come to the end of *Conquering Obesity, Conquering Mountains: 6 Steps to Fail-Proof, Sustainable Weight Loss and a Healthy Lifestyle Through a Holistic System*, you now have the tools, mindset, and strategies to make lasting changes in your life. Throughout this book, we've explored how to approach weight loss and wellness through a holistic, sustainable system. The journey to healthier living is not just about losing weight—it's about transforming your entire lifestyle and mindset to create long-term success.

We addressed why most weight loss efforts fail, examining common barriers such as unrealistic expectations, unsustainable habits, and a lack of long-term commitment. We introduced the importance of a holistic, sustainable approach—one that integrates your mental, physical, and emotional well-being. By focusing on balance, persistence, and realistic goals, you set the stage for lasting change.

Chapter 1, Cultivating a Positive Mindset for Weight Loss Success emphasized the critical role that mindset plays in achieving your goals. A positive, growth-oriented mindset is essential for overcoming the inevitable challenges that come with weight loss.

In *Chapter 2, Managing Stress for Sustainable Weight Loss*, we explored how stress is a powerful force that can derail progress. Learning to manage it effectively is a key step in ensuring your efforts are sustainable.

Chapter 3, Optimizing Time Management for Weight Loss offered practical strategies to help you prioritize your health goals despite the demands of daily life. It focused on making your health a priority and finding balance within your busy routine.

Chapter 4, The 8 Essential Elements of Healthy Living provided a framework to guide your daily actions, ensuring that you address all aspects of your life, from nutrition and exercise to sleep and relationships.

In *Chapter 5, The 6-Step System for Continuous Improvement in Weight Loss*, we introduced a proven method—a detailed, actionable roadmap—to ensure that your efforts are constantly evolving. By following the PDCA (Plan-Do-Check-Act) cycle and performing regular SWOT analysis on your weight loss journey, you can continue to refine your approach, ensuring that every step you take brings you closer to your long-term goals. With real-life examples and practical tips, this chapter helped you understand how to apply the system in your daily routine, making it easier to track progress, evaluate your efforts, and adjust as necessary.

Chapter 6, Building Habits That Stick focused on the importance of habit formation. Lasting health and weight loss success depend on building habits that are manageable, sustainable, and in alignment with your long-term vision. We explored tools to stay accountable and motivated, as well as strategies for overcoming plateaus and setbacks along the way.

Finally, *Chapter 7, Achieving Success and Wellness Simultaneously* defines success and wellness in your journey. It started with a Life Assessment, offering an honest inventory of your current state, including physical health, mental well-being, relationships, and overall satisfaction. The chapter also covered setting meaningful goals and time management, helping you maximize efficiency. It highlighted nurturing a supportive network and prioritizing self-care for a balanced lifestyle.

Now, as you look ahead to your journey, it's important to apply everything you've learned in this book. Each chapter has built upon the last, providing you with a comprehensive framework to tackle your weight loss and health goals holistically. The journey will require patience, consistency, and perseverance, but the tools and strategies outlined in this book have prepared you to tackle obstacles, stay focused, and succeed in your long-term wellness journey.

As you continue to implement the principles outlined in *Conquering Obesity, Conquering Mountains*, you will not only achieve your weight loss goals but also build a healthy lifestyle that supports your overall well-being. Whether it's through cultivating a positive mindset, managing stress, optimizing your time, or forming sustainable habits, you have everything you need to create lasting change.

In your path ahead, know that every step you take brings you closer to the healthiest, happiest version of yourself. Stay committed, stay focused, and keep applying these principles with confidence. Your journey to a healthier life is just beginning—and with the right mindset and approach, there's nothing stopping you from reaching the mountaintop of your health goals.

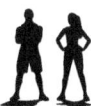

EPILOGUE: BEYOND THE SCALE – EMBRACING LIFELONG WELLNESS

As you reflect on your journey through *Conquering Obesity, Conquering Mountains*, it's important to remember that the true measure of success is not found solely in the numbers on the scale. While weight loss is a significant milestone, it's only one part of a much larger picture. The ultimate goal is to embrace a lifestyle that fosters health, balance, and happiness in all areas of your life.

Lifelong wellness goes beyond physical appearance—it's about feeling vibrant, energetic, and strong in your body, mind, and spirit. It's about finding joy in the process, not just in the outcome. By adopting the holistic approach we've discussed throughout this book, you've already taken the first steps toward creating a lasting, sustainable lifestyle that will serve you well for years to come.

When you continue on your wellness journey, it's essential to remember that setbacks and challenges are not failures, but opportunities for growth. Life will always present obstacles, but the tools you've learned in this book—like the 6-Step Cycle, the importance of accountability, and the power of habit formation— will keep you on track. Every challenge you face is simply another step toward building resilience and mastering the skills you need to thrive.

Think of this book as the beginning of a lifelong journey. With every small, intentional step, you are creating a future where your health and wellness are not just goals, but a way of life. You've already proven to yourself that you have the strength, commitment, and mindset to succeed. And now, as you move beyond the scale, you have the ability to embrace a future of well-being, vitality, and joy— one that reflects the best version of yourself.

Remember, the road to wellness is not about perfection. It's about progress, consistency, and self-compassion. Celebrate each victory along the way, no matter how small, and always be kind to yourself in moments of challenge. You are worthy of the health, happiness, and fulfillment that comes with lifelong wellness.

The journey doesn't end here—it's just the beginning. Keep embracing the principles that have guided you so far, and continue to step forward with confidence, knowing that with every new habit you form, every obstacle you overcome, and every positive change you make, you are shaping the life you deserve.

Now, go ahead and conquer your next mountain—because with your commitment, determination, and the tools you've gained, there's no limit to what you can achieve. Here's to your lifelong journey of health, wellness, and happiness.

"Climb the mountain not to plant your flag, but to embrace the challenge, enjoy the air and behold the view. Climb it so you can see the world, not so the world can see you."

—David McCullough Jr.

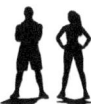

APPENDIX

Healthy Recipes and Meal Ideas

Every culture has its own healthy and delicious dishes. The challenge is not the lack of healthy options but rather our tendency to focus on the wrong ones, often struggling to control portion sizes and the frequency of meals. For a successful and sustainable journey, you do not need to adopt a Mediterranean diet or something entirely foreign to you. In fact, sticking to the types of food you already enjoy and are familiar with can significantly increase your chances of long-term success.

You do not need to buy salmon, eat avocados, or switch to expensive ingredients that may feel out of reach. While these foods are often marketed as "healthy essentials," they are not the only path to a healthier lifestyle. Instead, focus on meals and ingredients that are already part of your culture—foods that are affordable, accessible, and comforting.

Here are some examples to inspire you. Stick to your roots, embrace what is already part of your daily life, and make small adjustments to create a long-term, healthy lifestyle.

Chinese Dishes

1. **Steamed Fish with Ginger and Scallions**

Ingredients:

- 200g white fish fillets (e.g., tilapia or cod)
- 1-inch piece of ginger (thinly sliced)
- 2 scallions (sliced into strips)
- 2 tsp soy sauce (low sodium)
- 1 tsp sesame oil
- ½ tsp white pepper
- 1 tsp cooking oil
- Optional: A few cilantro sprigs for garnish

Directions:

1. Rinse the fish fillets and pat them dry. Sprinkle with white pepper.

2. Place the fish on a heatproof plate suitable for steaming. Spread ginger slices on top.

3. Steam the fish over boiling water for 7–10 minutes, depending on thickness, until fully cooked.

4. Heat the sesame oil and cooking oil in a pan. Once hot, add the scallions and stir-fry for 10 seconds.

5. Remove the fish from the steamer. Drizzle soy sauce over it and pour the hot scallion oil on top.

6. Garnish with cilantro and serve immediately with steamed rice

or vegetables.

Why It Works:

- Steaming: Retains nutrients without adding unhealthy fats.

- Fish: Low-calorie protein that supports muscle growth.

- Ginger and scallions: Add flavor without extra calories.

2. **Vegetable and Egg Stir-Fried Rice**

Ingredients:

- 1 cup cooked brown rice (preferably day-old)

- 1 egg (beaten)

- ½ cup mixed vegetables (e.g., carrots, peas, corn)

- 2 garlic cloves (minced)

- 2 tsp soy sauce (low sodium)

- 1 tsp sesame oil

- 1 tsp cooking oil

- Optional: Chili flakes for spice

Directions:

1. Heat the cooking oil in a non-stick pan or wok. Add garlic and stir-fry until fragrant.

2. Add the mixed vegetables and stir-fry for 2–3 minutes until tender.

3. Push the vegetables to the side of the pan and pour in the

beaten egg. Scramble until cooked.

4. Add the cooked rice to the pan. Toss everything together and drizzle with soy sauce and sesame oil.

5. Cook for another 2–3 minutes, ensuring the rice is evenly coated. Serve hot.

Why It Works:

- Brown rice: A whole grain that provides long-lasting energy.

- Egg: A budget-friendly source of high-quality protein.

- Vegetables: Add vitamins, minerals, and fiber while keeping the dish low-calorie.

Indian Dishes

3. Egg Bhurji (Indian Scrambled Eggs)

Ingredients:

- 3 eggs

- 1 onion (chopped)

- 1 tomato (chopped)

- 1 green chili (optional)

- ½ tsp turmeric powder

- ½ tsp cumin seeds

- Salt and pepper to taste

- 1 tsp oil

Directions:

1. Heat oil in a pan. Add cumin seeds and let them splutter.

2. Add onions and sauté until translucent. Add tomatoes, green chilies, and turmeric.

3. Crack eggs into the pan and stir continuously until they scramble.

4. Season with salt and pepper and serve hot.

Why It Works:

- High-protein, low-carb breakfast option that boosts satiety and metabolism.

4. **Oats Upma (Healthy Breakfast)**

Ingredients:

- 1 cup rolled oats

- ½ cup chopped vegetables (carrot, peas, beans)

- 1 onion (chopped)

- 1 green chili (chopped)

- 1 tsp mustard seeds

- 1 tsp urad dal (optional)

- 8-10 curry leaves

- 1 tbsp oil (or use spray oil)

- ½ tsp turmeric powder

- Salt to taste

- Coriander leaves (for garnish)

- Lemon juice (optional)

Directions:

1. Dry roast the oats in a pan for 2-3 minutes until slightly golden. Set aside.

2. Heat oil in a pan, add mustard seeds, curry leaves, and urad dal.

3. Add chopped onions and green chili. Sauté until onions are soft.

4. Add the chopped vegetables, turmeric, and salt. Cover and cook for 5 minutes.

5. Add roasted oats and mix well with the vegetables.

6. Pour in ½ cup hot water and stir continuously until oats absorb the water.

7. Turn off the heat, garnish with coriander leaves and squeeze lemon juice.

Why It Works:

- Oats: Rich in soluble fiber, which keeps you full longer and supports digestion.

- Vegetables: Add volume with minimal calories and increase fiber intake.

- Minimal Oil: Reduces fat content while keeping the dish flavorful.

Malay Dishes

5. **Ayam Percik (Spicy Roasted Chicken)**

Ayam Percik is a flavorful and aromatic grilled chicken dish popular in Malaysia. The chicken is marinated in a rich blend of spices and coconut milk, then grilled to perfection, resulting in tender, juicy meat with a smoky char.

Ingredients:

- **For the Chicken:**
  - 1 whole chicken (about 1.5 kg), cut into 8 pieces
  - 2 stalks lemongrass, bruised
  - 3 kaffir lime leaves, torn
  - 1 inch ginger, sliced
  - 1 teaspoon turmeric powder
  - 1 teaspoon salt
  - 1/2 teaspoon black pepper
- **For the Spice Paste:**
  - 6 shallots, peeled
  - 4 cloves garlic, peeled
  - 2 inches ginger, peeled and sliced
  - 1 inch galangal (lengkuas), peeled and sliced (optional, adds a sharper flavor)
  - 3 red chilies (or to taste)

- o 1 tablespoon chili powder (optional, for extra heat)

- o 1 teaspoon turmeric powder

- o 1/2 teaspoon coriander powder

- o 1/2 teaspoon cumin powder

- o 2 tablespoons vegetable oil

- o 1 tablespoon tamarind pulp, mixed with 2 tablespoons water

- o 1 cup thick coconut milk

- o Salt and sugar to taste

Directions:

1. **Prepare the Chicken:** Clean and pat the chicken dry. Make a few slashes in the thicker parts of the chicken pieces to help the marinade penetrate.

2. **Make the Spice Paste:** Blend all the spice paste ingredients (except oil, tamarind water, coconut milk, salt, and sugar) into a smooth paste.

3. **Cook the Spice Paste:** Heat oil in a pan. Fry the spice paste over medium heat until fragrant and it starts to darken in color (about 8-10 minutes). Add the tamarind water, salt, and sugar. Cook for another 5 minutes, stirring occasionally. Taste and adjust seasonings.

4. **Marinate the Chicken:** Add the coconut milk to the spice paste and bring to a simmer. Pour this marinade over the chicken pieces, ensuring they are well coated. Marinate for at least 30 minutes, or longer for a more intense flavor (ideally, marinate in the refrigerator for a few hours or overnight).

5. **Grill the Chicken:**

- **Charcoal Grill:** Prepare a medium-hot fire. Grill the chicken, turning occasionally and basting with the marinade, until cooked through and slightly charred (about 20-30 minutes).

- **Grill Pan:** Heat the pan over medium-high heat. Grill the chicken, turning occasionally and basting with marinade, until cooked through (about 15-20 minutes).

- **Oven:** Preheat oven to 200°C (400°F). Place the chicken on a baking sheet lined with foil. Bake for 30-40 minutes, or until cooked through, basting occasionally with the marinade.

6. **Serve:** Serve the Ayam Percik hot, garnished with lime wedges and extra sambal (chili sauce) if desired. It's delicious with plain rice, nasi kerabu, or ketupat (rice cakes).

Tips:

- Lemongrass and Lime Leaves: You can also stuff some of the lemongrass and lime leaves under the skin of the chicken for extra flavor.

- Spiciness: Adjust the amount of chili in the spice paste to your preference.

- Coconut Milk: Use thick coconut milk for a richer flavor.

- Basting: Basting the chicken with the marinade while grilling helps keep it moist and adds flavor.

6. Sayur Lodeh (Creamy Vegetable Stew)

Sayur Lodeh is a comforting and flavorful vegetable stew cooked in a creamy coconut milk broth. It's a popular dish in Malaysia and

Indonesia, and each family often has their own unique version. Here's a basic recipe that you can adapt to your liking:

Ingredients:

- **For the Spice Paste:**
  - 5 shallots, peeled
  - 3 cloves garlic, peeled
  - 1 inch ginger, peeled and sliced
  - 1 inch galangal (lengkuas), peeled and sliced (optional, adds a sharper flavor)
  - 2 red chilies (or to taste)
  - 1 teaspoon turmeric powder
  - 1/2 teaspoon coriander powder
  - 1/2 teaspoon cumin powder
  - 2 tablespoons dried shrimp, soaked in hot water and drained
  - 2 tablespoons vegetable oil

- **For the Stew:**
  - 1 cup thick coconut milk
  - 3 cups water
  - 1 tablespoon tamarind pulp, mixed with 2 tablespoons water
  - 1 teaspoon salt, or to taste
  - 1/2 teaspoon sugar, or to taste

- o Vegetables (choose a variety, about 1 kg total):

  - 1 cup long beans, cut into 2-inch lengths

  - 1 cup cabbage, roughly chopped

  - 1 cup carrots, peeled and cut into chunks

  - 1 cup potatoes, peeled and cut into chunks

  - 1 cup green beans, trimmed and cut into 2-inch lengths

  - 1 cup eggplant, cut into chunks

  - 1 cup chayote (sengkuang), peeled and cut into chunks

  - Tofu puffs or tempeh, fried until golden brown (optional)

Directions:

1. **Make the Spice Paste:** Blend all the spice paste ingredients into a smooth paste.

2. **Cook the Spice Paste:** Heat oil in a large pot or wok. Fry the spice paste over medium heat until fragrant and it starts to darken in color (about 8-10 minutes).

3. **Make the Stew:** Add water and tamarind water to the pot. Bring to a boil. Add the vegetables that take longer to cook, such as carrots and potatoes. Simmer for about 10 minutes, or until slightly softened.

4. **Add Remaining Ingredients:** Add the remaining vegetables, salt, and sugar. Simmer for another 5-10 minutes, or until all the vegetables are tender but still hold their shape.

5. **Add Coconut Milk:** Reduce the heat to low. Stir in the coconut milk. Simmer for a few minutes to allow the flavors to meld. Do not boil vigorously after adding the coconut milk, as it may curdle.

6. **Serve:** Serve Sayur Lodeh hot with steamed rice. You can garnish with fried shallots and fresh chilies if desired.

Tips and Variations:

- Vegetable Choices: Feel free to use other vegetables you like, such as cauliflower, broccoli, or corn.

- Spiciness: Adjust the amount of chili in the spice paste to your preference.

- Tofu and Tempeh: Adding fried tofu puffs or tempeh adds protein and texture to the stew.

- Leftovers: Sayur Lodeh tastes even better the next day as the flavors develop further.

- Serving Suggestions: Sayur Lodeh is often served with lontong (compressed rice cakes), nasi impit (pressed rice), or ketupat (rice cakes).

Western Dishes

7. Quinoa Salad with Lemon Vinaigrette

Ingredients:

- ½ cup quinoa (cooked as per package instructions)

- ½ cup cherry tomatoes (halved)

- ½ cucumber (diced)

- ¼ cup red onion (finely chopped)

- 2 tbsp feta cheese (crumbled, optional)

- 1 tbsp olive oil

- 1 tbsp lemon juice

- ½ tsp Dijon mustard

- Salt and pepper to taste

- Fresh parsley or mint (for garnish)

Directions:

1. Cook the quinoa according to the package instructions and let it cool.

2. In a large bowl, combine the cherry tomatoes, cucumber, red onion, and cooled quinoa.

3. In a small bowl, whisk together olive oil, lemon juice, Dijon mustard, salt, and pepper to make the vinaigrette.

4. Pour the vinaigrette over the quinoa mixture and toss well to combine.

5. Sprinkle feta cheese and garnish with fresh parsley or mint before serving.

Why It Works:

- Quinoa: A complete protein rich in fiber and minerals.

- Vegetables: Low-calorie additions that enhance taste and nutrition.

- Lemon vinaigrette: A healthy, flavorful dressing with no added sugars.

Tracking Tools and Resources

To help you stay on track with your weight loss and wellness goals, here are some practical tools and resources to make tracking easier and more effective.

1. **Food and Activity Log**

Keeping a daily log of your food and activity can significantly increase awareness of your habits and help you make more mindful choices. Use a journal or an app to track:

- **Meals and Snacks:** Write down what you eat, portion sizes, and when you eat. This helps identify patterns in your eating habits.

- **Exercise:** Record the type of activity, duration, and intensity. It will help you see improvements and stay motivated.

- **Mood and Energy Levels:** Tracking your emotional state and energy throughout the day helps you see how food and exercise impact your well-being.

2. **Progress Tracker**

Track measurable progress such as:

- **Weight and Measurements:** Track your weight, body measurements (waist, hips, thighs, etc.), and body fat percentage to monitor changes over time.

- **Fitness Goals:** Track your fitness milestones, such as the amount of weight lifted, distance run, or flexibility improvements.

- **Health Metrics:** Monitor your blood pressure, blood sugar levels, and other key health metrics with the guidance of a healthcare professional.

3. **SMART Goal Setting Template**

To ensure that your goals are clear, measurable, and achievable, use the SMART framework:

- **Specific:** Define exactly what you want to achieve.

- **Measurable:** Track your progress with specific numbers or milestones.

- **Achievable:** Set a realistic goal based on your current abilities and lifestyle.

- **Relevant:** Make sure the goal aligns with your overall health and wellness objectives.

- **Time-bound:** Set a deadline or time frame for achieving the goal.

4. **Mobile Apps for Weight Loss and Wellness**

- **MyFitnessPal:** Track food intake, exercise, and progress with this popular app.

- **Strava:** Great for tracking outdoor activities like running, cycling, or walking.

- **Headspace:** A meditation app to help manage stress, which is essential for sustainable weight loss.

- **Fitbit:** Wearable tech to track steps, sleep, and exercise, providing a holistic view of your health.

5. **Support and Accountability Resources**

- **Online Communities and Forums:** Find groups or forums (like Reddit, Facebook, or specific wellness sites) for weight loss and wellness support.

- **Accountability Partners:** Connect with a friend, coach, or family member who can offer encouragement and keep you accountable.

- **Health Coaches:** Consider working with a certified health coach to personalize your weight loss journey and stay on track.

These resources and tools will help you stay on top of your goals and track your progress, making it easier to stay motivated and maintain momentum. Whether you're logging meals, tracking exercise, or reflecting on your achievements, these tools are here to support you every step of the way as you continue on your journey to a healthier, happier life.

www.ingramcontent.com/pod-product-compliance
Lightning Source LLC
Chambersburg PA
CBHW061739270326
41928CB00011B/2296